What They Don't Teach You In Dental School

Everything you need to know about setting up and running a dental practice

by Jeffrey V. Anzalone, DDS
with Halle Eavelyn

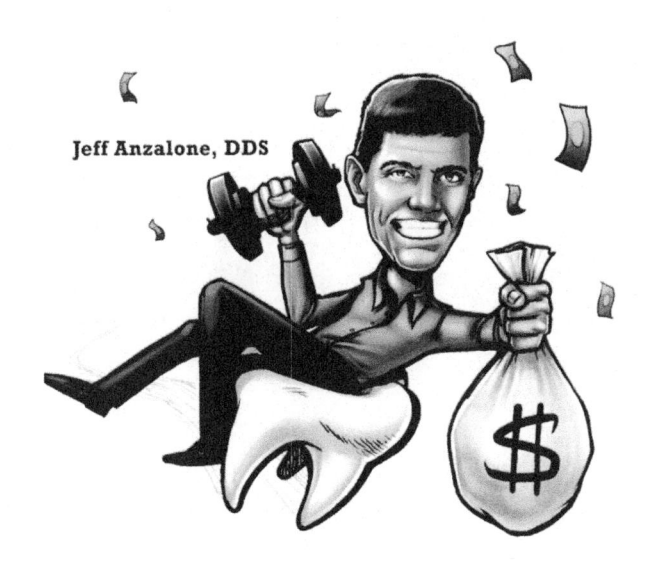

Dedication

Thanks to all the dentists who contributed stories and their personal experiences to this book: Dr. Ron, Dr. Gina, and especially to my dear friend, Dr. Brian, for his invaluable contribution.

I feel fortunate that I was blessed enough to find a great network of people who have helped me on my journey down the path of dentistry: Dr. Phil Rothermel, Dr. Chuck Anzalone (my uncle), Dr. Mike Nolan, and Dr. Lance Donald.

For my beautiful wife Rebekah — I can't live without you and I couldn't have done it without you.

All of the websites and businesses I speak of in this book are ones that I use or trust and I am in no way being compensated for recommending them.

TABLE OF CONTENTS

Introduction

PART I: BASICS FOR SETTING UP A PRACTICE 8

Chapter 1: The Making of a Dentist 9

Chapter 2: The World According to Dave Ramsey 17

Chapter 3: The Fledgling Dentist 19

Chapter 4: What Every Dental School Didn't Teach You 24

              Accounting and Business Structures 24

              Taxes 26

              Bank Accounts 27

              Managing Your Finances 28

              Payroll, Payroll Taxes and Deductions 30

Chapter 5: Setting Up Your Practice 33

              Insurance 34

              Occupational License 38

              Labor Laws 39

Chapter 6: The Backbone of Your New Practice 41

              Practice Management Software 41

              Chartless Systems 42

              Dental Practice Consultants 44

              Employee Policy Manuals 45

              Job Descriptions & Systems 46

              Money Safety 47

Chapter 7: Equipping Your Office 48

              Dental Equipment 48

	Computers & Back-up Systems	50
	Office Supplies	52
	Office Telephones	53
	Credit Card Terminals	55
	Medical Waste Disposal	55

PART II: MARKETING THE PRACTICE 56

Chapter 8:	Getting the Word Out	57
	Literature	57
	Marketing You	58
	Websites	58
	SEO and Keywords	59
	Social Media	60
	Newsletters	60
Chapter 9:	It's All About the Patients... Right?	63
Chapter 10:	No-Resistance Selling *Getting a Yes! for Treatment*	72
Chapter 11:	How to Become THE Authority Dental Practice in Your Town	81
Chapter 12:	The Rest of What They Didn't Teach You	88
	First Impressions	88
	Testimonials	89
	Making Patients Comfortable	89
	Continuing Education	90
	My Final Piece of Advice	91
Bonus Chapter	Dr. Brian Evans Story	92
Afterword:	Taking the Next Step	99

Introduction

I have a confession to make. When I wrote the first edition of this book, I was mad. Why, you ask? Dental school. That's right, dental school. To be a little more specific, I was angry because of the really important stuff that was not in our curriculum. Certainly our dental schools should be able to squeeze in classes regarding:

- starting a practice from scratch;
- running the day-to-day operations;
- hiring, firing, and training employees;
- top ways to get patients to say "yes" to treatment recommendations;
- internal and external marketing; and
- how to answer the phones properly to get patients in your chair.

Literally all the important stuff listed above is conveniently left out of the dental school curriculum. This made me really angry, which sparked me to write a book in the first place. But now, after several years of my book's original release, and receiving reviews that the book was too basic, I decided to write an update.

Times change and dental practices have to keep up with these changes—or go out of business. I have become an avid student of everything regarding marketing. I absolutely love it. Do you know what I love even more? Teaching it.

Nothing makes me happier than assisting dentists with their unique practice problems and getting positive results to help them eradicate their issues.

I honestly had NO IDEA that the original version of this book would be so popular! I was even more surprised by the number of young dentists who are constantly searching for the type of information I teach.

Let me tell you a few things that have changed for me personally since the first edition was published. When you hear what has happened in my life and practice, I think you will get excited about what's to come in your future.

The original version of this book was the first book project I had ever undertaken. I must admit that the entire process of writing, editing, designing, printing, and publishing was a lot to take on by myself. It took well over a year (much longer than I expected). Fast forward to the present, and I'm working on my fifth book, a process that now takes me only a couple of months. This is no different from when you and I were in dental school. At first it may have taken us 2-1/2 hours to prepare a tooth for a crown from start to finish, but after doing several such procedures, the time to complete the treatment decreased considerably.

In 2013, I applied for and was accepted as one of the finalists for Marketer of the Year at the Glazer-Kennedy (GKIC) SuperConference (gkic.com). This is one of the largest, if not the largest marketing conferences for small to large businesses. The experience of preparing for and giving my presentation in front of close to 1,000 individuals was amazing. The numerous people I've met while networking at GKIC events have helped shape and grow my practice to what it is today. If not for them, I would not have started a separate company to help dentists with their practice issues and problems from a dental professional's standpoint. They were also instrumental in encouraging me to write books and to use them to leverage my businesses (more on this subject later).

Many of you reached out to me after reading the original version of this book. You gave me mixed reviews and requested more in-depth information. After looking back over the first edition, I now realize it was very "basic." That said, I wanted to give students and young dentists the basics first. They needed to crawl before they could learn to walk.

If you are reading one of my books for the first time, congratulations! You are in for information overload. One of my colleagues, who is also an author, recommended that I add only a chapter or two to this new edition, but there was too much information in my brain to stop there! I've added about 25 percent more information than was in the first edition—and I am keeping the price the same. As long as you find value in what I have to say, I'm going to keep saying it.

I would love your feedback on this new, updated version. Please send your comments to **drjeffreyanzalone@gmail.com** or fax to **318.998.2503**.

Also, if you enjoy this updated version, I'd love for you to share the love with others. Simply search for this book on Amazon and leave your review.

The past reviews are what I use to add content to future versions so I can continue to make this book more relevant and provide the information dentists want most.

Now, let's begin ...

PART I:
BASICS FOR SETTING UP A PRACTICE

Chapter 1
The Making of a Dentist

I can still remember the phone call as if it were yesterday. I was in my final month of a Periodontics Residency at LSU and couldn't wait to get out and make some real money. I was planning on moving back to my hometown of Monroe, Louisiana, so I could join a group dental practice. I had been talking to the Senior Partner periodically throughout my residency and he had a job waiting for me.

I called him about a month before school ended with my muchanticipated graduation date, and was abruptly punched in the gut with the news that I was not needed any more. Just like that, my future dreams of an easy life in an established practice were knocked out of me. I went from elated to terrified in the space of a few moments. I had just purchased my first home (after renting for eight years) and I had a wife in the next room, comforting my crying two-month-old baby. What was I supposed to do now?

At this crucial moment of my fledgling career, I suddenly realized I had been solely dependent on the group's knowledge to teach me the business side of dentistry, and now I didn't have a clue how to proceed without them. I remember walking into our bathroom after the call ended, shutting the door and sitting down on top of the toilet. I asked God to help me. I was as scared as I have ever been in my life. I had just learned firsthand that life is constantly knocking us down and it's our job to keep getting up and moving forward. (I think I heard that line in a Rocky movie?) The Chinese have a wonderful old saying about it, too. Fall down seven times, get up eight. Either way you prefer, the message is the same. It was up to me to get through this if I was going to have a successful practice.

I had spent most of my life in Monroe, only leaving it to go off to college and pursue my dream of becoming a dentist. Monroe is a medium-sized town of over 50,000. Located in the northeast part of Louisiana, it has a generous supply of southern hospitality and plenty of hunting and fishing to keep folks occupied. I grew up with loving parents and a brother who I had the usual bickering with, but who was really one of my best friends.

When I was seven years old, a friend and I were playing with matches in a neighbor's back yard. You know how your momma always told you not to play with matches? Or pour gas on a fire? Well, apparently we hadn't learned those lessons yet, because my friend and I lit a little fire, then he doused it in gasoline. The resulting conflagration gave me second and third degree burns on my legs, and put me in the hospital for the next two weeks, where I had to undergo multiple surgeries. Luckily, I saw such compassion and care from the doctors and nurses every day, that it was a huge life lesson for me. By the time I was released from the hospital, I knew I wanted to be some kind of doctor. My friend didn't fare as well. Though he escaped uninjured from the fire, his dad beat the crap out of him and grounded him for the whole summer.

At twelve years old, I started a small lawn service, which kept growing. When I went off to college, I gave the business to my brother, but it had already helped me deal with customer service, and learn to pay for tools. It was also a real-life lesson in how to run a business, even on a small scale. My brother ran it for another six years. My small lawn-care business started a lifelong desire to be an entrepreneur. I was always told I was pretty mature when I was a kid, but I could see as a teenager that the other kids were dependent on their parents for their allowances, but I had the pride that came along with earning my own money.

My dad taught me by example – he never sat me down and told me not to use credit cards, but he always paid everything in cash. If we didn't have the cash, we just went without. I guess my work ethic came from way back – my grandfather started his hardware store in Monroe in 1941, and my father started in the store at 21; he just celebrated 40 years in his store. While this business mindset surely shaped my character as a child, it's not a necessity—you can still learn some business basics for your own practice, no matter what kind of background you come from.

Sports have always been a big part of my life. Playing baseball, basketball, tennis and football helped shaped my character, humbled me at times and taught me discipline and my strict work ethic. The sports programs after school were very structured. Honestly, I worked the hardest in Little League, where we were taught to stay at the top of the lineup. When I was playing, I noticed something interesting: my friends whose dads were surgeons mostly missed their kids' games, but my friends with dentists for dads, like my good friend, Dr. Mike Nolan, always made it to their sons' events.

I decided I wanted something where parenting came first and my career came second. My uncle, Chuck Anzalone, also played a huge role in my decision to select dentistry as my profession. As I was growing up, he introduced me to a hobby I now share with my own boys today: bass fishing. My uncle has four kids, and seeing him enjoy the type of lifestyle that provided a good living for them, plus allowed him time to do the things he enjoyed, helped solidify my decision to go into dentistry.

In middle school and high school, our teamwork and discipline continued because of these early lessons in structure. In 1992, I graduated from Neville High School, which is known for its football program. Now, my boys, Brooks and Benton, my dad and I look forward to spending our Friday nights together in the fall watching the Neville Tigers play ball under the lights.

I graduated from Northeast Louisiana University on a partial scholarship, and my folks ponied up the rest. Then I entered LSU Dental School in 1996, which I paid for on my own, mostly through loans but also partly funded by my business. If you're reading this while you're still in high school or in your first part of college, good for you for getting an early start! Just know that starting part-time work in high school and continuing that during college and medical or dental school will help to offset the enormous costs of college. Between us, my wife (who is my dental hygienist) and I took out nearly $200,000 in school loans. The average today for two people is closer to $300,000, and we were above average in our need to borrow. What you will require is up to you, but it's safe to say that the costs will only go up.

After graduation, we got on a thirty-year-plan to repay, which would have meant we were responsible for those student loans longer than for raising our kids! We didn't want the debt hanging over our heads forever, so we aggressively paid the loans off within seven years. Finding the motivation to do so was very arduous, as there's no tangible reward, like when you buy house and get to live in it. But saving $200,000 is reward enough. Do anything you can to get your loans reduced quickly, such as joining the military or a dental practice, or taking an extra job— it's worth it not to have a huge debt hanging over your head.

Free Bonus: My friend Dr. Brian's personal story of going into the military to pay for his dental school is a Special Appendix at the end of this book.

While I was at dental school, I met the love of my life. Once a month, the school hosted a TGIF party with a local band and some food and drinks. This one particular evening, I had enjoyed a beer or two and was hanging out with my friends, when I saw Rebekah for the first time. Rebekah was so beautiful, I couldn't help but stare at her. I nudged my friend Brent and pointed her out. Brent laughed. He dared me to go over and try to talk to her. I was wearing a pair of overalls and a cowboy hat; Rebekah told me many years later that I had looked so ridiculous coming across the room to say, "Howdy."

I invited her out, and despite the funny outfit, she gave me her number. While it took a whole bunch of dates for Rebekah to know I was the one for her, I knew she was the one for me that very first night. Rebekah was attending Dental Hygiene school when we met. We got married soon after I graduated from dental school, and she supported us financially for three years while I attended my residency. Pretty crazy, huh? She went to school for a lot less time, and got out into the job market much sooner and was able to make a good living at it. It almost makes you want to reconsider all that extra work, huh?

Sometimes things happen for a reason. After all these years, I know why I didn't pass my state board exam the first time around; I had more to learn. The State Boards are taken near graduation and not offered again until the following year, so when I didn't pass, my Uncle Chuck (the dentist) came through in the clutch for me once again. After making some phone calls to several influential people, he was able to help me acquire a position at the VA in Biloxi, Miss., and continue my training with a one-year general practice residency. As you can imagine, I was devastated. I had been looking forward to my graduation and working in Crowley, La., with my uncle, but sometimes things happen to send you down a different road.

Initially, living in Biloxi was difficult. I had never before lived in a place where I didn't know a soul. Luckily I found a couple, Dr. Philip and Barbara Rothermel, who helped me navigate this difficult time in my residency. Dr. Philip has always been an avid golfer, and he was also one of the staff dentists at the VA. His crown and bridge work was flawless.

I always thought once they graduated and no instructor was looking over their shoulders, dentists would tend to relax and not try to make everything "perfect." If this is true, then Dr. Phil was an exception.

Looking back, that one year I spent in Biloxi was one of the best years of my life. I fished a couple of days a week, and Dr. Phil inspired me to take up golf again. We spent countless hours after work on the driving range and the golf course trying to hone my skills. The many hours he spent me with in the clinic and at the course helped make my one year away from home seem not so bad after all.

Dr. Philip was also instrumental in critiquing my work to the point that it became almost as good as his, which allowed me to pass the state board on my second exam. Uncle Chuck had the courage and enough faith in me to allow me to treat my cousin Katie during my state board exam. Though working on a relative instead of a stranger was more comfortable for me during this stressful time, it was much easier because I was very wellprepared.

To this day, Dr. Phil and I stay in touch and he helps keep me on the right path—not only concerning dentistry, but also life in general. I believe it is very important to find a mentor early on in your career, someone you can trust and look up to and who always has the time to stop whatever he or she is doing to help you along the way.

During my time at the VA in Biloxi, I began to show interest in periodontal surgery, so I applied and was accepted to attend a three-year residency in Periodontics at Louisiana State University. Contacting local dentists regarding starting up a scratch practice was a high priority at the end of my residency. A recurring statement was, "Try to start up practicing with little to no debt. Rent before you buy. Purchase used equipment or better yet, rent someone else's equipment." I took these statements to heart and can honestly say that I implemented all of them initially. This was huge! The whole time, I kept thinking, "How can I obtain money to buy and equip a building?" Taking out more loans was out of the question.

Looking back, now that I am in a solo practice and don't have to take orders from anyone, I can see that not being able to practice in a group was one of the best things that has ever happened to me. I guess the phrase, "Things don't happen to you but for you," is true! At first, I was devastated, and when I confessed to Rebekah that my cushy new position in an existing practice was gone, it was one of the hardest things I'd ever done, even though I had her support and love. It taught me that honesty was the best thing I could give to my life partner, just as the Senior Partner of the dental practice had been honest with me. That's something I have carried with me always, and it's a characteristic I can highly recommend. Whether business is up or down, people will always respect your integrity.

As often happens in small geographic locales, word spread quickly throughout my hometown about my experience. A wonderful endodontist, Dr Lance Donald, contacted me to say that he was in the process of renovating a large vacant office. Would I be interested in renting space? The idea of my own practice sounded great, and here was the perfect place to begin it, but I still had no idea how to go about the nuts and bolts of creating my own business.

Possibly even more terrified at the prospect of being successful than I was of failing, I began scrambling to find as much online information I could. I also networked daily with other dental professionals regarding starting a practice from scratch. While there is some information out there, a lot of it is biased towards the companies that produce the material. For instance, if you perform an online search for: "starting a dental practice from scratch," the majority of the hits will be from loan companies, banks, dental CPAs and dental brokers. They're all offering you their information and explaining in articles and on web pages why you should do business with them. As I was just coming out of dental school, taking out more loans was the last thing I wanted to do.

I wasn't sure what to do yet, but my Internet searches already had my gut instinct shouting, "no more debt!" I had to find some way to go into practice myself without incurring more loans, but still procure the necessary equipment I needed to work. You've never heard of a modern dentist practicing with a pair of pliers and a hand mirror, have you? Well, I didn't intend to be the first. I would keep looking, to ensure that I had the best chance to succeed. My family's future was at stake, and I couldn't let them down.

Chapter 2
The World According to Dave Ramsey

Several years before I graduated, I began listening to financial guru Dave Ramsey, and to this day, I still follow his principles. His basic program creates a sound structure of basic, smart financial advice that I would recommend to anyone. I'm outlining the big ideas here, but I urge you to explore his sensible suggestions in detail. You can find out more about him and his financial teachings at www.daveramsey.com (and no, I didn't get paid to say this).

Dave's ideas resonated with me completely when I first heard him speak. After all, I could relate. Dave started from nothing, and by the time he was 26 had a net worth of a little over a million dollars and was making $250,000 a year. Except for the million dollar net worth, a beginning dentist is in a similar circumstance, and I liked the idea that I could grow my net worth, too, instead of going into debt.

Dave was a big part of my thought process during my transition from student to practitioner. If not for his guidance, I would have immediately picked out new dental equipment, instruments, and computers that I thought I had to have to practice. I also would have taken out more loans. I was already in over a hundred thousand dollars in student loan debt, and had taken out a mortgage before earning one penny! I could not imagine borrowing another three to four hundred thousand dollars to buy dental equipment and a building to start up my practice. I would have been close to three-quarters of a million in debt, nearly the exact inverse of Dave's net worth! The very thought put knots in my stomach.

Unfortunately, this is what happens to many of the students graduating from professional schools today. We want it all and we want it now. Dave calls this "doc-itis." What would our grandparents have done? I can assure you your grandma and grandpa would not have bought anything that they couldn't pay for. Why? Well, just a couple of generations ago, there was no such thing as credit, unless it was the weekly tab you ran up at the local bar or general store.

Charge cards, where you could run up a balance and pay it off in full once a month, weren't even started until the 1940s, when a business man American Express echoed Diner's Club in the late 1950s with a card for entertainment and travel expenses. This was followed by the first "revolving credit" account, the basis of today's credit cards, by Bank of America. By the late-70s, this BankAmericard had become Visa, and MasterCharge had renamed itself MasterCard. The credit boom was on. Today, over two billion credit cards are in circulation, most in the West, where our consumer society tells us to buy it now and pay for it later.

The backlash has been the recent recession, which has brought the type of philosophy Dave Ramsey teaches to the fore.

Dave has Seven Baby Steps to Financial Peace, which he outlines in full on his website (www.daveramsey.com) These include starting an emergency fund of just $1000, smart and easy ways to pay off your debt, and what to do with your money once you have retired your debt (but still have many working years of your career ahead of you).

By following Dave's simple and logical steps, and from the lessons I learned along the way, I was personally able to retire over a half-million dollars in debt much faster than originally estimated, plus open my practice, and start raking in the cash. And I'll have my house paid off in full in the next three years, too; a total of just ten years instead of fifteen or thirty. As a new doctor or dentist, you are getting the benefit of my experience, without having to make the mistakes I did.named McNamara started the idea of a "diner's club" for restaurants.

Chapter 3
The Fledgling Dentist

After graduating from dental school, I began working with my first partner, Dr. Lance, out of his two-operatory building. He was remodeling his office, and when the remodel took 5-6 months longer than expected, it gave me time to learn the ropes of practicing dentistry.

First, I started networking with potential referring dentists. I would show up and do a meet and greet with whoever was in the office, being especially nice to the front office staff members who would be referring me to their bosses, and who could help me get a foot in the door. Beginning specialty dentists have been known to bring in gift certificates, deliver lunch to a whole dental office, show up with baskets of flowers and cookies, and in general act like they have nothing better to do than press gifts on the established office. Which, really, you don't. If you are a dental specialist, these people will be the lifeline of your new business.

If you're not a specialist, you can still piggyback off of existing businesses by partnering or associating with an existing practice or chain. I know of a few dentists who have even bought out an older dentist's patient list, office, or practice when he or she was ready to retire.

For example, Dr. Gina, a dentist practicing in the LA area, went to UCLA Dental School, and when she wanted to strike out on her own, bought the client list and charts from a retiring dentist. He wanted someone he liked to take over the patients, so once he found Dr. Gina, he was willing to sell her the list for a very reasonable price. She estimates that she made around nine times that cost in revenue, all before building her own practice up.

I also worked part-time with a national denture chain, performing surgeries for their patients. Working for dental chains part-time is a great way to supplement your income while starting out, because dental students can graduate and begin working with great benefits, without acquiring more debt. If you're not specializing, this is a great way to acquire patients. I have a feeling that dental chains and large group dental practices will continue to grow, since they have strong brands and marketing that ensures a steady supply of patients.

Other dentists will choose to go into a group practice, where they can work on existing patients as their own. Again using Dr. Gina's experience, when she was in group practice, she got 40% of her revenues, and the practice paid all expenses and salaries. She also paid just 40% of the lab bills. Today, in a high-tech office, overhead in a specialty like Periodontics will eat at least 50% of your revenues, and in general dentistry can be as high as 70-80%, so remember that when you are choosing your career.

As a new dentist, my friend, Dr. Ron, drove one day a week to an oral surgery job sixty miles away. The revenue coming in helped to pay down his overhead as he established his practice. Dr. Ron kept that job for three years so that he wouldn't have to accrue additional debt. His recommendation is that you take a side job at least a day a week; I think you should work as much as you need to in order to stay out of debt your first few years in practice. It can mean being able to retire years earlier.

For the next two years with Dr. Lance, I worked at my personal office until noon, then with the denture chain during each afternoon. I was slowly acquiring referral patients from the dentists I was visiting, and eventually, I realized that my own practice was large enough to begin full-time.

In February 2006, we moved into the new location and I began to begin to observe how to manage a practice. I was still marketing to other dentists for more referrals and hiring staff. This was where dental school really fell short for me. I knew nothing about creating and setting up an office! My biggest initial mistakes were not having systems in place, and not knowing how to hire employees or train them. I had no employee handbook. That means we had no cell phone policy, Internet policy, or job assignments. If something didn't get done, staff would just say, "It wasn't my job." Everyday systems, such as walking a patient in and out, or who would take out the trash or clean the bathroom, were mass confusion for the first few years. Meanwhile, I was learning as I went. I made at least a hundred mistakes that could have been avoided.

For example, I used to hire and fire everyone myself, with no input from the rest of my staff. When my receptionist quit unexpectedly, I hired someone who was experienced in office reception; basically, she looked good on paper. Unfortunately, after the initial interview, she didn't smile, and she wasn't friendly or happy. The rest of my staff hated her. She lasted a month.

Now, I cut way down on my turnover by hiring only friendly, happy people my staff loves, and letting my existing team approve them. Once I interview the potential candidate, I let my staff interview them and take them to lunch. I even subject them to a semi-formal personality test. I can train someone to be my assistant so long as they are friendly, happy, and a team player. It's been amazing to see the difference in my staff now that I follow these simple rules.

Due to my lack of practice (and practical) knowledge, I elected to work the first two-and-a-half years as an associate on a collection percentage. This worked very well because I did not have to worry about managing a business or taking out loans and could focus on building my practice. In my opinion, this is the way to go.

Other dentists, I admit, have gone the loan route, and it's cost them.

I strongly believe that, as a new dentist, you should consider joining a dental chain or existing practice and really pay attention to what goes on with not only the clinical side but also the business side of the practice. Perhaps you are raring to go and start your own dental practice; I know I was. If you want to be a successful dentist, how many hours a week do you want to spend mastering the learning curve of running a small business? Or learning operations and marketing without any background or role models? Both in paying off debt and acquiring knowledge, this will be an enormous part of how quickly you succeed in your early years, not just on paper but inside your own head and in the reality of your accounting books.

However, note that many practices can be quite expensive to buy into if you intend to partner. My friend Dr. Ron looked into it, and realized that (assuming he leased space instead of buying) he could build his practice twice over for the same cost as to buy into an existing practice. Don't be afraid to comparison shop, and remember to think strategically when it comes to your future. It's easier to run the numbers both ways and compare, than jump into something and regret it later as you become more educated.

The more I worked, the more I realized that the hardest part was what I knew nothing about! I didn't have a clue how to hire or fire someone, how to deal with insurance companies, or which insurance policies were the best. I didn't know how to properly submit patient information for reimbursement, which meant I spent a lot of time redoing forms and delaying my payments. (Now we have standardized forms.) I didn't know how – or when – to file my taxes.

Figure out what works best for you. For example, most dentists (including my first partner), followed this system: we would tell patients what treatment was required, and we would check to see what their insurance would cover. Once the insurance company's coverage was established, the patient would make up the difference. But what I didn't know is that many insurance companies would ask us to submit more information before paying on a claim. Sometimes, they would refuse to pay, long after the patient had already paid their anticipated portion of the bill. When we went back to the patient, they would rightfully say, "You told me it would only be $500," leaving us with the rest of the bill. It made our office look bad, going back to ask for more money after they thought their bill was settled.

Then a woman asked to have her tooth removed, and after the service, told the receptionist she had left her money in her car. She went to her car to "get her purse" and never came back, leaving us with the bill! This happened not just once, but twice!

So I came up with a new system. I would ask patients to put down 20% of the estimated cost to schedule the treatment, then the remainder would be due the day of treatment. If the patient had insurance, we would file everything for them, but they would be the one who got reimbursed by the insurance and waited for their money, not me.

I was worried that by switching to the new system I might offend people or lose patients, but it's actually been great, and we stopped losing money! I've recommended this system to other dentists I work with, and it's worked great for them, too.

As I became more comfortable with dental procedures and began picking up speed, I tried to spend more time observing the administrative part of the business. The first thing I realized is that even the receptionist knew a lot more than I did, and that there was a whole portion of my education missing. My mind was overwhelmed with the knowledge that we never received a business education in school, and I was determined to learn everything I needed to know as quickly as possible. In the next chapter, you'll learn the low-level details that personally saved my bacon when I went into practice for myself.

Chapter 4
What Every Dental School Didn't Teach You

This next chapter and much of the rest of my book offer hardcore, detailed business advice. Though I think it's all perfectly useful and will help you out a lot, I have to make the disclaimer that I'm a dentist, same as you, and not an accountant, CPA, or attorney (nor do play one on TV). The rules may be different in your state, province, or region. Always consult with your own business professionals, as I did when setting up my own practice.

In their respective schools, other dentists I know got one lecture, or one class about the business of being a dentist. No one taught any of us that we would be small business owners, that we would be managing people, hiring & firing. We were taught to prevent disease and be excellent technicians. As far as I'm concerned, they left out the most important parts.

To make my transition from dental associate to being my own boss, I gave myself six months to prepare. I informed my mentor, Dr. Donald, that I wanted to begin paying my own bills and employees myself and split the overhead with him in the meantime. This was a great way to leave the nest without actually going. I had the advantage of an experienced, watchful eye to help me, yet I was able to function as if I were already on my own. As always in business, make sure that you are courteous and give your employer plenty of time before making changes or leaving.

Accounting and Business Structures
Before seeing patients, find an accountant you feel like you can really work with. I kept hearing the same accountant's name come up when I polled several dentists about which accountant to use. I met with the accountant and he instructed me to form an LLC, or Limited Liability Company.

An LLC is one of the most flexible business structures, as it can be either a partnership or a corporation for tax purposes. It's also gained a great deal of traction as the preferred type of corporate structure for small businesses, as it's also one of the least expensive to create and maintain, and the structure which requires the least amount of record keeping. Never co-mingle your personal and business funds in any structure, of course, but especially avoid doing so in an LLC.

The government treats an LLC as a "pass-through entity," which the income of the entity passes through to you and the other members of your LLC. If you're the only LLC member, the IRS treats the company as a "disregarded entity," so you would report your income on Schedule C of your personal tax return. If your LLC has multiple members, then it's considered a partnership by the IRS, and you or your accountant file your income under an IRS Form 1065. Then each LLC partner gets a Form K-1 reporting a share of the LLC's income (or loss) according to the portion of the LLC that person owns (e.g., 30% ownership, 30% of the taxable income) which that member then pays as tax.

When you form the LLC, your accountant can make a one-time election to have you taxed as a corporation; either a C or S Corp (see below).

The other types of entity are:

Sole proprietorship — a nightmare for taxes since your business is in essence taxed as an individual person S-Corp — one of the least understood and often most inaccurate classifications of entity. In the case of an S-Corp, income and loss passes through to the members.

C-corp — which is what almost all Fortune 500 companies use as their corporate structure. In a C-corp, the company pays taxes on all income before distributing to members, and then each member pays tax on the distributions or dividends the company gives them.

Partnership — which you might also want to consider as a structure, as it's very similar to an LLC.

A lot of accountants who work with small business owners suggest an LLC taxed as an S-corporation. While this structure gives you the tax benefits of an S-corporation (and its accompanying self-employment tax savings), you get the simplicity and easy record keeping of an LLC. Just remember to keep up with your meeting books and your annual meeting, and don't co-mingle your funds, so that if you are ever sued, the other side won't be able to "pierce the corporate veil," which basically means they can't come after your hard-won assets to satisfy any judgment in a lawsuit.

An attorney can perform the paperwork for you or you can also do it on your particular state's Secretary of State website or www.uslegalforms.com. Some accountants may want you to form a specific type of corporation, and you can't change the type of corporate entity once it's set up, so it's vital that you start with finding an accountant.

Taxes

After forming your corporation, you will need a Federal Tax ID number. Also known as an Employer Identification Number or EIN), this is the ID number assigned solely to your business by the IRS. Your tax ID number is used to identify your business to several federal agencies responsible for the regulation of business. You can contact your nearest Local IRS Field Office, call the IRS Business and Specialty Tax Hotline at 1-800-829-4933, or obtain one online in about 15 minutes. Visit **http:// www.irs.gov/ businesses/small/article/0,,id=102767,00.html** to read all about EIN numbers, then click the link to get one online during their business hours. More than likely your accountant will obtain your EIN number for you.

Any business offering services or products that are taxed in any way must get a federal tax ID number. If your state taxes personal services, or if you are required to collect sales taxes on your sales, you also need a federal tax ID number. All the government forms required for your business tax and entity filings will require either a Social Security number (if you are a sole proprietorship) or a tax ID number.

As you start your practice, you should immediately begin paying use tax, which is a sales tax substitute. All states that have a sales tax also impose a use tax to minimize unfair competition between sales made in-state and those made out-of-state. The use tax rate is the same as the sales tax rate. The Louisiana use tax is calculated at the rate of 8%. This 8% rate, which includes 4% to be distributed by the Department of Revenue to local governments, is in lieu of the actual local rate in effect in your area, and is payable regardless of whether the actual combined state and local rate in your area is equal to, higher than, or lower than 8%.

Keep up with your accountant, keep up with your taxes, so that you don't try to pay at the end of the year and get hit with a large tax bill all at once. Your accountant will set up payments to be made either monthly or quarterly. What we do is keep a folder of all the invoices received that are not charged sales tax. Copies of the invoices are given to the accountant on a quarterly basis to calculate and submit the payment to the state.

Bank Accounts

Once your accountant is in place, your corporation formed and a tax ID number, and you have opened a use tax account, it's time to find a bank and open a business checking account. A small local bank is likely to provide you with better personal service and refer local community members to you as you build a long-term relationship with them. On the other hand, you need to examine your own expected financial needs first.

If you like doing a lot of your banking online, all the large banks have mobile apps and websites that allow you to transfer money between your accounts, view all your transactions up-to-the-minute, and include fraud prevention alerts by text that keep you completely informed. So decide what's important to you in how you will bank, and choose your business bank accordingly.

You will need to provide them with your Tax ID number and name of your business, your corporation's name. More than likely it will be your name, John Doe, D.D.S, LLC.

While you are working for someone else, it's a good rule of thumb to put aside at least a third of what you make into a bank account designated for your taxes (usually as an independent contractor you'll make around 35-40% of collections). People often think that their taxes were taken out, but now, as an IRS class 1099 employee, you will be responsible for your own taxes. Use another bank account so you don't mix money, and even open it at another bank so you're not tempted to touch it.

Despite Dave Ramsey's philosophy about never buying anything on credit, I feel safer about ordering supplies with a credit card. If a mistake is made the company has not already accessed my checking account and taken the withdrawal, and with many credit cards, you are offered extra protection or a longer insurance period. If you think you may have trouble or are not disciplined enough to pay your balance off every month, I suggest sticking with a debit card instead.

I have both business credit and debit card accounts. You will need your Tax ID number when you open either account.

Managing Your Finances
When you open your checking account, I highly recommend ordering 3-part voucher checks like the one in Figure A, on the following page.

Figure A

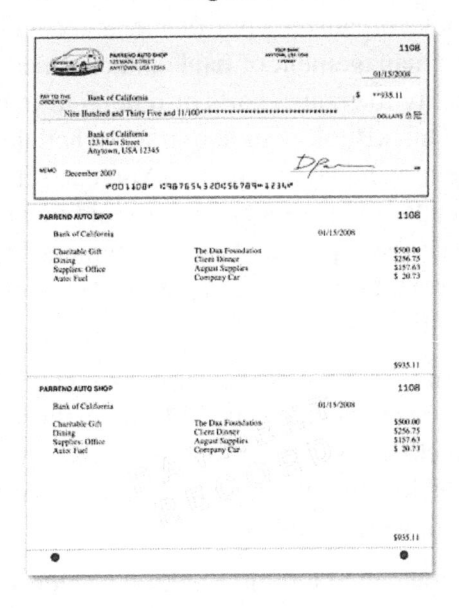

These checks are run through your printer, which allows you to keep a record of your purchases. For instance, when I pay a bill with an invoice, I take the middle and bottom section of the check and staple it to the invoice. I have a file cabinet, and one of my files is called Business Checks (one per year, with the year written right on the folder). All of the paid invoices go in here. This will help keep you organized as you pay numerous bills per month.

The way bills are paid and tracked is a vital part of your successful business. Sounds boring, but getting this system in place can make you more money as you time your bills, avoid late payments, and even request better terms with vendors by showing a strong credit history. Having an appropriate bill-pay software program will allow you and your accountant to keep track of where all the money is going for supplies, expenses, taxes, employees, etc.

I really like using Intuit's QuickBooks software for my business. QuickBooks organizes your financial accounts in one place. It allows management of bank and credit card accounts and has the ability to create charts or reports to track money in each account. QuickBooks can help track scheduled bills or any payment made to vendors or patients. You can set up recurring payments if needed. This tool can help avoid delayed transactions or in some cases, penalty for late payments. QuickBooks' payroll management option tracks payments to employees and can help you with filing taxes.

I started out using QuickBooks because my accountant recommended it. Your accountant can provide you with software to transfer the QuickBooks files between you, such as the RAS Client Tool, which allows me to send data for the accountant to review while still working on the data from my office.

There is a section called Online Banking Center that allows you to set up an electronic connection to your business checking account and your business credit or debit card accounts. You can upload the transaction information either manually or automatically, instead of typing in the information by hand, saving valuable time — your own!

Payroll, Payroll Taxes and Deductions
Another great feature about QuickBooks is the Liability Payments Center. Your accountant will calculate the different taxes you will have to pay (payroll, Federal, State, etc) and then post them in the Liability Payment Center. When you access this screen, you will see a list of the different taxes, the date in which they are due, and the amount to pay. You simply write checks or pay online for each of these by the due date. The website to pay online is: https://www.eftps.gov/eftps/direct/EftpsHome.page

A Form 941, or Employer's Quarterly Federal Tax Form, is the form used to report employment taxes, withholding amounts, deposit amounts, and amounts due to the IRS. The amount that is put in each time will be calculated after you run your payroll.

I was mystified about running payroll and was told by some other dentists that I needed a payroll service to pay my employees. With QuickBooks, payroll is simple. Your accountant will set up your employees in the employee section of QuickBooks and input the calculation for all the different taxes to be withheld each pay period. Taxes to be taken out will be Federal, Social Security, Medicare and the withholding State tax. You will give each new employee an L-4 and W-4 tax form, and they determine the amount of taxes to be withheld from each paycheck. Then you give the forms to your accountant.

Here's a quick primer on payroll. First, calculate how many hours the employees have worked. I pay my employees every other week (fairly standard practice, but you can also pay twice a month, or even weekly). The hours can be calculated from a simple time clock, whatever dental practice management software you are using, or a cool product I recently purchased when my employees were constantly forgetting to clock in or out, the TS100 Biometric Fingerprint System. http://lathem.com/ products/automated-systems/ts100-biometric-fingerprint-system.aspx)

The device uses fingerprint technology to identify and clock in and out of the system. Your personnel simply place a finger on a scanner and are recognized within seconds. This also prevents employees from clocking each other in or out.

Simply print off the timesheets for the dates of the pay period and enter the hours in QuickBooks. You enter the date when the pay period ends, type in the hours worked, and the taxes are automatically taken out of the check. Perform this operation for all employees, then all their checks can be printed at once.

QuickBooks offers great support, and you should not be afraid to also utilize your accountant for any technical questions you may have.

If you offer a retirement plan for yourself and your employees — and I believe you should give back to the staff which is supporting your successful business by offering this important perk to them — the deduction can also be set up by the accountant to be automatically included each month as well. The amount to put in the accounts each month will also be placed in the Liability Payment section along with the amount to match per employee.

For instance, I use a Simple IRA from Vanguard. I have been doing this from the time I began practicing, and three of my four employees currently contribute to the plan.

Every month, I log into the Vanguard Small Business website, select each employee that contributes, and type the amount to be deducted from their check and the amount to match as well. As I mentioned, the amounts will already be provided for you from your accountant and then you simply fill in the blanks.

The IRA account can be linked directly to your business checking account so the transfer of the money monthly will literally take seconds to perform. The Simple IRA limits for 2012 are $11,500 per person annually. If you are married and your spouse works with you, you can contribute $11,500 per year each with up to a 3% match of your salary. This is a great way to begin saving money until all your debts are paid.

After becoming debt-free, you will probably want to switch to a different retirement vehicle that allows you to save more, to give you the most benefits in tax savings. This is where you should seek the advice of your accountant and financial advisor.

Chapter 5
Setting Up Your Practice

As a dental associate with an existing office, you can now see you have several advantages. One that I haven't mentioned is that you can practice up until the day it is time to for you to move into your new building as your own boss. When I struck out on my own, I was lucky enough to move into a building previously occupied by another dentist.

I currently practice out of a 1750 square-foot office with three operatories (treatment rooms). I recently read an article in a dental magazine, a first-person experience of a new dentist who had started his practice from scratch. He began renting in a new strip mall, paying over $4000 per month in rent alone, and had also purchased every type of new technology imaginable. If I owed that type of rent and equipment loans every month, I wouldn't be able to sleep at night. This critical level of stress is perfectly avoidable, and by reading and following the advice in this book, you won't have to worry about it at all.

Should you rent, purchase or build? This is a great question and depending on your unique situation, could be answered in a number of different ways.

I am all about renting or buying a building instead of using new construction, as I do not believe a new dentist should spend large amounts of money building and equipping an office from scratch. When I moved into my building, the landlord gave me an option to buy at anytime in the future. I rented for a little over a year to make sure that I liked the layout, location, etc. After a year of renting, I bought the building and updated it; but first, I saved up for the down payment and then paid for the entire remodel job in milestones as it was being completed. I can't find a commercial lot to build an office in my area for what I paid for the building and remodel job. My strong suggestion is to buy on location first, then remodel the place to your liking. Even if you have to hire an architect and a designer in addition to a contractor, underneath the facelift, most buildings are pretty much the same.

Insurance

Once you are ready to begin your search for a property, locate a reputable local insurance agent. You will need coverage for the building you buy or rent, in case of fire or a catastrophic event.

Coverage will pay for building a new building plus equipping it as well. You also need other policies in case a patient is injured in your office, a staff member is injured (workman's comp), possibly flood insurance, etc. These insurance policies should be in place before you begin treating patients. Consult with someone you can trust, who will teach you what you need in your area and why.

The insurance information below outlines plans from the American Dental Association (ADA). Great-West Life is my insurance group, which is affiliated with the ADA. They have numerous plans to choose from and I have not been able to find cheaper rates. Of course, you should choose the program, agent, and insurance that works best for you.

Term Life

I recommend level term life insurance if you are married or have children. Twenty to twenty-five year term limits should be sufficient to cover if something should happen to you, and give you peace of mind knowing that your family will be taken care of. A good rule of thumb for the amount of coverage is 10x your annual income. For example, if you make $150,000 per year then obtain $150,000 x 10, or $1.5 million in coverage. The beneficiary should be instructed to invest the amount and live off the dividends. Don't take this part for granted. If the beneficiary lives off the principal, they will spend all the money and have none left to live on, and most people don't think ahead like that!

Disability Insurance

This insurance is a must, because you never know when something may happen to prohibit you from working. I injured my elbow playing basketball in a church recreational league, when I collided with another player who hit me directly on the funny bone. My arm was numb for a day and sore for a couple more. I was not able to work the next day, which scared me to the point of purchasing this insurance, when I realized that an injury could occur that was out of my control.

When you first purchase disability insurance, you will only be able to buy a limited amount of coverage. For me, that number was $5000/month initially, then coverage can be increased annually upon renewal. The Plan includes a true "own occupation" definition of disability that can pay benefits all the way to age 65. If you become totally disabled from your specialized area of dentistry, you'll get full benefits, even if you choose to work in another area of dentistry or if you choose to enter a new profession.

Office Overhead Expense Plan

This is something that I just recently purchased. If you are an associate you probably don't need it. This plan pays up to $25,000 or more of the monthly expenses to run a practice, such as rent, payroll, taxes, supplies, etc. It's nice to know that your office and staff will be taken care of if you are unable to work.

Health Insurance

Health insurance is a must these days. A good website to check policies is www.ehealthinsurance.com. A good rule of thumb is to choose a policy that offers a Health Savings Account (HSA) option.

An HSA is a major medical policy with a high deductible and low premium. Make sure the policy you choose is HSA-compatible.

You can save up to around 70% on your premiums, as you are saving money that can be used tax-free on medical expenses. The amount saved in the account rolls over from year to year, which allows those savings to gain interest. Money can be withdrawn tax and penalty-free whenever it's needed for medical expenses. If the money is used for anything else, you pay a penalty and taxes. The money in the account must be used for medical, dental and vision care.

Malpractice Insurance
Malpractice insurance is a necessity, but don't make the mistake I did and purchase from the reps who come into your school before graduation. They will insist that if insurance isn't purchased at that moment, rates will skyrocket! I fell for this, but cancelled a few months later after finding other options, (which happened to be a lot cheaper). My recommendation is to either ask local dentists which companies they use, or use your favorite search engine.

There are a couple of policy options available regarding malpractice insurance. An "Occurrence Policy" responds to a loss, if the policy is in force at the time a medical incident occurs. A "Claims-Made Policy" responds to a loss if a policy is in force at the time a claim is reported. Below is a detailed explanation of both.

Occurrence Policy
When you purchase an Occurrence Policy, the premium you paid up front will cover all claims for malpractice during that policy year. No additional premium is required if you cancel your policy.

For example:
A medical practitioner purchases an Occurrence Policy from a carrier for 2005. The insured decides not to renew for 2006. The carrier is presented with a claim in 2007 for surgery the practitioner performed in 2005. The company will defend the

practitioner because the incident occurred during the policy period of 2005, during which the practitioner was insured.

However, if the same medical practitioner had performed the surgery in 2006, the carrier would not provide coverage for the practitioner, because the incident occurred after the policy period ended.

Claims-Made Policy
The main difference between Occurrence coverage and Claims-Made coverage is that the event insured under a Claims-Made Policy is covered regardless of when the occurrence took place.

When Claims-Made coverage is initially purchased, the premium charged will be lower than premiums collected for comparable Occurrence Policies. The premium charged for the Claims-Made coverage is made based upon the possibility that a claim will be made during the year of the premium charge. Claims resulting from professional services are not usually reported during the first year; therefore, the first year's Claims-Made premium is significantly lower than the following years' premiums.

This stair-stepping of premium continues for five years until you reach a mature premium. At that point, assuming there are no rate increases, your premium remains stable and you pay the same premium every year thereafter, with one significant exception. That exception occurs when you cancel your policy. It is the Reporting Endorsement.

Reporting Endorsement, or "tail"
Occurrence Policies do not require extended Reporting Endorsements (tails) if coverage is discontinued. This is because if the insured event occurs during the policy's period, then coverage under the Occurrence Policy applies regardless of when the claim is made.

Claims-Made Policies, however, do require the purchase of tails if the coverage is discontinued. This is because the policy only covers claims that are made during the policy's period. Future claims may arise and be first reported after the termination date of your Claims-Made Policy. A tail provides insurance for covered losses arising after your retroactive date, and reported after your policy's termination date.

Before purchasing any insurance policy, check with your state dental association. Most states have a list of companies and vendors that they endorse, which give members a discount.

Occupational license
To practice many occupations, from a hairdresser to a dentist, you are required to hold a license and be certified in any state you work in. If you move, you must obtain a new license. You may contact your local city government to obtain information or go to http://www.govspot.com/state, select your state, then select Professional and Occupational Licensing found under the Licenses, Permits and Records section. Upon applying for a license, an inspector will be sent out, usually from the local Fire Department, to make you sure the building is up to code and fire extinguishers are in place. We use a local oxygen supply company to provide the extinguishers and the yearly maintenance (and they can service your oxygen and nitrous oxide tanks periodically as well).

After you pass the building inspection, an Occupational License is issued. Next, contact the local State Board of Dentistry and let them know you are changing addresses and ask if any inspections are required. If you perform IV sedation, you must obtain an onsite inspection, usually from an oral surgeon affiliated with the board and one other board member. Every state is different so it is very important to check and make sure you are following the correct procedures.

In my state of Louisiana, dentists performing conscious sedation must have a personal and building permit. This covers all types of sedation, including nitrous oxide. These licenses, along with your dental license, labor laws, and malpractice insurance, should be posted on an office bulletin board for easy access.

Labor Laws

Wikipedia says that labor law (or "employment" law) is "the body of laws, administrative rulings, and precedents which address the legal rights of, and restrictions on, working people and their organizations. As such, it mediates many aspects of the relationship between trade unions, employers and employees."

I recommend searching Google to obtain your state and federal labor law posters. State and federal laws impose numerous requirements and prohibitions on American businesses, but one of the most overlooked obligations is the responsibility to conspicuously display various government labor law posters in the workplace. The purpose of these labor law posters is to inform employees of their rights under applicable laws and provide information on how to report discrimination, wage and hour violations and other rights infringements to the government.

Occupational and Safety and Health Administration (or OSHA) safety programs and compliance kits can also be readily obtained online. OSHA regulations (both at the state and federal level) require employers to provide a safe and healthful workplace foremployees, reduce or eliminate recognized safety hazards, and comply with standards relating to specific work practices or conditions. OSHA compliance products can help businesses prevent injuries, protect workers, and avoid fines for noncompliance.

The General Duty Clause of the OSHA Act states that each employer "shall furnish to each of his employees employment and a place of employment which are free from recognized hazards

(29 USC654(a)) and comply with OSHA standards promulgated under the Act (29 USC 654(b))."

Violations of the OSHA Act or related OSHA standards can result in fines up to $7,000 per violation for non-serious and serious infractions. Willful and repeat violations can result in much higher fines, up to $70,000. So those posters are important as well as necessary.

So far we have our building in place, and have obtained licenses and insurances. Now we need to equip it!

Chapter 6
The Backbone of Your New Practice

Some of the most important parts of your new office are actually not physical equipment. They are computer software and your new staff.

Practice Management Software

First, your practice management software, the "brain" of the dental practice. I personally use PerioExec from DSN out of Washington State. They also have other programs for other specialties and for general dentistry.

Dentrix is a very popular practice management software for general dentists. If you begin your career as an associate, you should familiarize yourself with that particular practice's software.

Most practice management software utilizes the Internet for updates and electronically filing insurance. You may be thinking to yourself, "How do I electronically file insurance?" Do not fret. Your practice management program that is purchased will have this built into the software. You will receive instruction during initial training on how to perform this.

A nice inexpensive add-on to your practice management software is NEA FastAttach (http://www.nea-fast.com). This is a program that is downloadable which allows dental providers to transmit supporting documentation for electronically filed claims. Documentation such as: periodontal charting, patient notes, digital x-rays, letters to insurance companies on why treatment is needed, etc. are documents that can be sent electronically that cuts down on time and also allows the provider to keep track of what is sent with each claim.

Occasionally, dental insurance companies will send letters claiming that certain documents are missing and need to be provided before the claim can be processed such as x-rays or periodontal charting. If the documents were sent electronically, an electronic claim number can be provided to the insurance company as proof that the document was sent. This helps not only the dentist but the patient, in that the whole process is much smoother and faster.

It will take several months to get the hang of the software and then you should begin making written recommendations about how to make the program better.

For instance, you may want to add a different feature to the program or you may not like how something is worded. Most of these computer companies will take your recommendations seriously and will usually change or modify the program. If you do not like the program you start out using, begin to look into other programs that suit your needs. The program should be user friendly for all your staff members, so make sure to ask your staff about their experiences as well. The software should also have the capability of being totally chartless.

Chartless Systems
I adamantly recommend starting off chartless if at all possible. Over the course of your dental career, you will save a huge amount of money by not having to buy charts, paper, filing cabinets or anything that has to do with paper charts. Don't forget ease of access, a hidden time waster when you have to look things up physically.

When I began my associateship, we used paper charts for the medical history page, financial policy page and HIPPA page. Once I branched out on my own, I began scanning all these forms into our computer system, thus eliminating the need for charts.

In our office, we have two main printers at the front desk to which all six of our computer stations are networked. I have my own personal computer and printer in my office. We have a flatbed scanner to scan all forms into the system and a signature keypad from Topaz software (www.topazsystems.com), for patients to sign consent forms after reading a laminated copy.

I contacted my practice management software company before purchasing the printers, scanners, and keypad and they gave me a list of accessory electronic equipment that work best with their software.

Most software is Microsoft Word-based for clinical progress notes, letters, etc. Initially, templates and forms will have to be set up and then placed in the system. This is very time consuming initially, and is a continuous work in progress, but it is easiest to do it up front when you have fewer patients and your practice is not yet thriving.

Examples of forms that we have in our system are: consent forms, HIPPA forms and financial forms, which can all be seen on our website, (http://www.anzaloneperiodontics.com).

Most software will have a notes or progress notes section for day-to-day patient entry. I initially set up templates for consults, exams, post ops, and every type of procedure that we perform. Here's the template we use in the office for extractions:

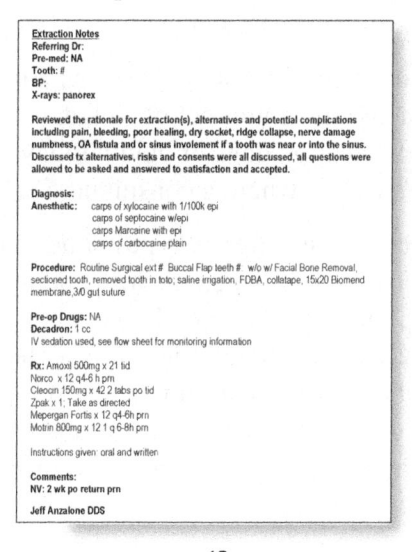

Extraction Notes
Referring Dr:
Pre-med: NA
Tooth: #
BP:
X-rays: panorex

Reviewed the rationale for extraction(s), alternatives and potential complications including pain, bleeding, poor healing, dry socket, ridge collapse, nerve damage numbness, OA fistula and or sinus involvement if a tooth was near or into the sinus. Discussed tx alternatives, risks and consents were all discussed, all questions were allowed to be asked and answered to satisfaction and accepted.

Diagnosis:
Anesthetic: carps of xylocaine with 1/100k epi
carps of septocaine w/epi
carps Marcaine with epi
carps of carbocaine plain

Procedure: Routine Surgical ext # Buccal Flap teeth # w/o w/ Facial Bone Removal, sectioned tooth, removed tooth in toto; saline irrigation, FDBA, collatape, 15x20 Biomend membrane,3/0 gut suture

Pre-op Drugs: NA
Decadron: 1 cc
IV sedation used, see flow sheet for monitoring information

Rx: Amoxil 500mg x 21 tid
Norco x 12 q4-6 h prn
Cleocin 150mg x 42 2 tabs po tid
Zpak x 1; Take as directed
Mepergan Fortis x 12 q4-6h prn
Motrin 800mg x 12 1 q 6-8h prn

Instructions given: oral and written

Comments:
NV: 2 wk po return prn

Jeff Anzalone DDS

As you can see, a lot of work goes into making these templates but saves a tremendous amount of time being able to just fill-in blanks when patients are treated. I obtain most of my patients through referrals from other dentists, and these templates also allow me to copy and paste into a Word document that I can then send as a letter to the referring dentist, advising them what treatment was performed on their patient.

The practice management software companies usually send someone to train you and your staff for a day or two. Have all staff members take good notes and start a group binder, because there will be numerous questions that will initially come up. Most of the companies charge a monthly or annual fee for support and upgrades, so help is just an email or phone call away.

Dental Practice Consultants
After I discontinued my associateship, I had two employees, a dental assistant and receptionist. They were used to working with me and the other dentist, but then I realized that nothing was written regarding office policies. What happens if someone quits or I need to hire an additional person? Consider hiring a practice consultant. I hired a group to come in for 2 days to observe my practice and put office management systems in place.

For instance, you are in the process of hiring a new employee and they ask you about the number of sick days (I personally don't have them), vacation days or paid holidays you offer? What do you do? This is where a consultant can help.

These types of consultants offer all types of helpful services ranging from assisting over the phone to spending time in the office. The group I used was Classic Practice Resources in Baton Rouge, LA (www.classicpractice.com). I informed them of my situation and told them I needed someone to come to the office, see how the practice was running, and give recommendations for putting systems into place. I wish I had hired them from day one!

I couldn't believe how much I didn't know or didn't have, that should have been implemented. They shadowed our office for two days, then on the second day sat down, first with me then with the entire staff, and made numerous recommendations.

Employee Policy Manuals
They also provided me with a generic office policy manual, which I customized regarding my specific practice. For example, I implemented a monthly collection bonus, and specified our policies for paid holidays, vacation time, etc. Now I had something for potential and present employees to reference if there were questions.

A policy manual also helps with new employees who are not performing well. If you have to let an employee go, you have your policies in writing and can point to why they are being let go: not following procedures, taking personal calls at the office, violating office Internet policy, etc. This really helps legally if a previous employee tries to file a complaint alleging they were fired unjustly.

The consultant can also provide generic consent forms, financial policy forms, HIPPA forms, etc. that can be modified for your practice. We have these forms on our website, so patients can print them at home and bring them to the office to be scanned into our system. We are currently adding an online registration function to the website, where a patient can fill out information and we will be notified via email when a new patient requests an appointment.

Most of the consultants can also provide you with information and forms regarding hiring new employees. Of course you can always take out an ad, but this is rarely the best way to find good staff. I tend to rely on word of mouth for potential employees or approach someone I interact with at a local establishment, such as a bank or restaurant, who I feel would be a good fit for my office.

The number one key to look for in hiring someone is his or her personality. Look for nice, happy people. You can teach anybody to do clerical work or dental assisting but you can't teach people to be kind. I've tried and trust me, it doesn't work.

I have a great staff right now, but I never know when someone may leave. Most of the forms consultants provide tend to be about how to structure an interview, and questions to ask the applicants. You can also obtain Employee Evaluation forms. You can implement these when you are doing quarterly (or at least annual) evaluations where you will also discuss strengths, weaknesses, and areas where the staff person can improve.

Potential employees must read your Employee Policy Manual first, then have them ask any questions regarding your policies. It's better to get possible problems out of the way before they begin work.

Job Descriptions & Systems
Once an employee is hired, you'll want to have systems in place regarding job descriptions. Most consultants can help with this by providing generic forms you can customize. For the first employees you hire, have them write down everything that they perform, step by step, in a notebook (which you can have typed up) or on a computer. After this is completed, future employees will be able to come in and perform all required tasks by following the documented procedures. The more detail, the better the list.Start with from the time they open the front door, turn off the alarm, turn on compressor, etc. to the time that the door is locked at the end of the day.

Once the system is created, try handing it over to another staff member to test and see if they are able to perform the duty correctly. Or bring your consultant back in to test the system. Keep adding more detail until you are satisfied that the task is being performed correctly with few outstanding questions. Then you will know your system is ready.

Money Safety

Office embezzlement is quite common, and a friend of mine had over $150K embezzled by a trusted staff person. I personally handle payroll, pay the bills, and file the employee retirement contributions. It's up to you how comfortable you feel doing this, but keeping your hands on your checkbook ensures that your money stays where it belongs. I spend around thirty minutes a week, now that my systems are in place, so this is time well spent ensuring my money is safe.

Most offices have petty cash. My staff keeps a hundred dollars in cash on hand, broken into different denominations. A friend suggested that on an occasional weekend I throw in some extra money, just to see what happened. When my receptionist came in and handed me my money back, wondering why there was extra money in the petty cash, I was especially gratified, and was able to prove to myself that my new receptionist was trustworthy.

I also make the bank deposits, and generally handle everything that has to do with money. Even if you choose to hand the day-to-day tasks over to your office manager or perhaps your accountant, you still need to be looking at your books each month.

Have your accountant run cash flow and income statements (the backbone of your financial docs) monthly, and then share those with you, going over them line-by-line until you are comfortable reading the reports. Make sure you also look at your profit and loss statements at least quarterly, since that can show you a pattern of your company's spending and achievements. Ask your accountant to help you by making suggestions as to where you can reduce your business expenses, but remember that he or she is not a dentist, so there may be large expenses that you need to maintain. You will make the final decisions on what's best for your growing practice.

Chapter 7
Equipping Your Office

I bought an existing building that had recently housed a dental practice, so I was also able to purchase their used equipment, which saved me tens of thousands of dollars. Buying used equipment from local dentists or on the Internet is a great way to start out in practice. You don't need state-of-the-art equipment to treat patients and make an income, no matter what the sales reps tell you. Remember that they are getting paid on commission. I'm not, and I have my own personal experience to share.

Dental Equipment
Whether it's purchasing equipment, software, or services, it's getting more expensive to be a dentist. Most of these products today aren't just bought once, they're maintained with a monthly fee you will pay for upgrades, maintenance, support, and/or training, so costs are ongoing and your overhead can naturally be quite high.

If you are planning on building an office, I highly recommend that you work with your local dental equipment representative in regards to equipment recommendations. I do not recommend new construction for the new dentist, for the reasons already outlined in previous chapters.

The best-case scenario would be renting an existing dental office, but that may not always be an option. If you begin your career as an associate, plan a timeline to move into your new office. This will help tremendously with regards to the financial aspect of the move, as you can save and begin to acquire the equipment that you will need. I began purchasing equipment each month, a year in advance of moving into my new location.

Always get multiple quotes from different vendors and let them know you are a new dentist starting up. You will be surprised by the amount of "new dentist" deals there are out there.

If you are buying new equipment, make sure that it has a warranty that does not begin until the day you begin using the equipment (as opposed to the day you buy it, perhaps months before you need it).

As I have said before, my strong recommendation is that you buy used equipment at first, with cash instead of on credit. If you purchase it through a company, you can probably get a warranty for it. I've bought mostly from individuals and have never bothered with a warranty, and I've also never had problems with the equipment I've purchased. It's up to you as to your level of comfort in this matter. Of course, it's likely that even if you had repair costs for used equipment, you would still come out ahead of buying new. When you start with used equipment, as your practice grows, little by little you can begin replacing older equipment with new equipment – which you also buy with cash, of course.

Your local dental rep can tour the building and help come up with a plan to equip the operatories and design the layout. If you are happy with the space you are currently using, by all means use the same layout. Talk to local dentists about the move and get names of local sub-contractors such as plumbers and electricians. These guys will come in handy if any renovations need to be performed.

I explained earlier about opening a business checking account with a local bank. If you do plan on taking out an equipment loan, most of the local banks will work with you personally and may not even require a business plan. Some of the equipment vendors offer financing in order to bypass a bank, but if you plan ahead then you can save enough money to pay cash for your equipment and office renovations.

I strongly recommend speaking with your accountant before purchasing any equipment, due to future tax projections and depreciation schedules. Also, the accountant will more than likely want a new LLC formed for the building if you're purchasing or doing new construction. This keeps the building separate from the dental practice and helps with liability issues and future taxes.

Computers

A computer system is one of the most important parts of your successful dental practice. A chartless office will usually consist of a server, a computer in each operatory, one in each doctor's office, and one or two in the front office.

Consider using a local computer company to build a system for you. I initially obtained a quote for an office full of name-brand computers for $20,000 but was able to get a local company build a system with more memory, and install it, for less than $10,000. However, the main reason for using a local company is customer service. If an issue comes up or something is not working, it's nice to have someone come to the office (usually the same day) for service instead of being put on hold with someone in a foreign country who will try to diagnose your problem over the phone.

Before having your system built, pick out your digital x-ray equipment. Most digital x-ray software and practice management software systems require a certain amount of memory to store images and data. We currently use Sirona for our sensors (#1 and #2 sensor) and a Sirona digital panorex. Sirona's software is called Sidexis and we obtained their data storage requirement specifications, then gave them to our computer tech to incorporate as he built the system.

There are numerous digital x-ray systems to choose from, so my advice is to try as many out as possible, preferably at a dental convention. Most of the time you can purchase the demonstration models for a hefty discount.

Have the local Internet representative from your practice management software meet with your computer tech to discuss networking the office. You can avoid a lot of headaches if you take care of this ahead of time.

Back-Up System

Have the computer technician recommend an automatic backup system using external hard drives. We currently use three external hard drives to back up all our office and financial information. One is left plugged into the computer, one is kept in our fire safe, and one is taken home.

Most servers have a back-up feature and the time of the actual back-up can be set any time. You'll want it to back your system up at night, when the office is shut down. Make sure your new back-up software is set to add to the old data daily instead of adding a full back-up file, thus saving lots of space on the hard drive and time for the back-up to complete.

The latest technology is backing up to the "Cloud, which means backing up online to a (usually unlimited) system that is housed at someone else's large storage facility." I recently read research stating that 50% of all tape backups cannot be recovered in full, due to handling errors. Most offices use tape, CD, or external hard drive back-up methods. These are all good, but if something physically happens to the back-up device or storage material, you lose your data.

An automated Cloud Back-up system like Dropbox, SugarSync, or Jungledisk is an ideal addition to your back-up needs. The backups will occur automatically over the Internet with little hassle. The data is encrypted to safeguard protected health information, maintaining a patient's privacy. We currently use Jungledisk and pay less than $10 a month.

Another cool feature is that you can install the back-up software on any computers you like, which means you can sync files and folders from all your computers, including tablets and smart phones, which means you have access to all these docs from your home (or the beach). If you alter a document on your office computer, it's automatically updated on your other computers, so long as the software is running with an Internet connection.

Computer Monitors
Computer monitors come in multiple sizes; make sure you purchase one large enough for you and your patient to view an xray or photo. Make sure the screen is mounted in a way that it can be moved in front of the patient but also against a wall, especially if the room is small. An expanding mounting arm can help with this. If the operatories are large enough, then two monitors can be set up, usually behind and in front of the patient.

Office Supplies
Most dental reps will have a list of practically everything routinely purchased in a practice, from sutures to paper points. This can help you ensure your new office is properly equipped. Keep an Excel or Word document of all supplies ordered, along with vendor phone numbers. Always ask for specials when ordering equipment and supplies; if none are available they may offer you free shipping instead.

If you associate initially, you can obtain their instrument and supply list. If you are happy with the office's setup and supplies, I suggest going room-to-room and writing down every instrument, supply, and, if possible, ordering information. For instance, in the sterilizing room, you could create an Excel spreadsheet that includes the make and model of the autoclave, the different sizes of autoclave bags, etc. Write down every single possible item ordered and take pictures of how the rooms are set up so that you don't have to rely on your memory when you are in your new space. I took pictures of the opened drawers and the insides of cabinets, too. You can laminate these pictures to educate new employees on setting up rooms and trays.

Most instrument vendors provide hefty discounts to the new dentist. Also, there's nothing wrong with using the instruments from your dental school days. I am still using some of the same instruments after twelve years. It's amazing how long an instrument will last if you take care of it and keep it sharpened.

Office Telephones
If the practice management software is the brains of the office, then the phones are the heart of the dental office, and deciding how many lines to have can be challenging. How many you get will perhaps determine the size of your practice (getting a busy signal will deter new patients, who may just move down to the next dentist on the list) so be sure to err on the side of "more than enough."

Our office started with one main phone line, a rollover line, and a fax line shared by the credit card and Care Credit (outside patient financing) terminal.

We now have four phones lines and a fax line (shared with credit card terminal and Care Credit terminal.) My recommendation is to start off with two lines, one rollover line, and one fax/credit card line. Just make sure there is room to add more lines if needed.

We recently consulted with Jay Geier's Scheduling Institute to train our staff how to properly answer the phone and schedule patients. They recorded and provided us with "mystery calls" received by our dental staff when answering phones.

It was a very eye-opening experience. On one call, my receptionist told the "mystery patient" who wanted her teeth cleaned, "Our office only cleans teeth when it's in conjunction with surgery."

I couldn't believe it!! After my blood pressure returned to normal, I had a talk with the entire staff to clear up any misconceptions about what we can and can't do. No telling how many new patients we were running off, but you learn from your mistakes. Obviously, this was well worth my time and investment.

Credit Card Terminals

Credit card terminals will be a must when setting up your front office. We purchased ours through FTS, Financial Transaction Services.

Every time a patient uses a credit or debit card for payment, you must pay the credit card company a percentage. Not only do they collect money from you, but also from the patient if they are late paying their bill. No wonder credit card companies make so much money!

Our office also recently purchased a device from FTS to verify checks. We used to receive a handful of checks that bounced every year. With the economy taking a downturn, we began receiving more and more of these, so we purchased a TeleCheck terminal.

When a patient presents a check to the receptionist, the check is authorized through a specially designed, secure TeleCheck system that captures banking information and the amount of the check. Once the check is approved, you'll receive a receipt of the electronic transaction to sign. When you sign the receipt, you get a copy for your records along with the check, which you can keep.

This has saved us in returned check fees that the bank charges, and also from having to contact patients days later who thought they paid their bill in full. However, I do not recommend purchasing this system unless you begin to have problems.

CareCredit
This is a great way to offer folks interest-free financing when they don't have insurance or can't pay everything all at once. CareCredit is exclusive for healthcare services and was started to help patients pay for medical implants; now they offer no-interest short-term financing, and low-interest longer-term financing.

Medical Waste Disposal
Before you start seeing patients, you need to hire a medical waste disposal service. Check your local state dental association's website for recommended medical waste disposal vendors.

We currently use Stericycle. The company you choose provides complete custody documentation, which is essential for accountability and regulatory compliance of bio-hazardous materials. They also provide all necessary containers in which you place contaminated sharps and other materials such as soiled gauze, patient bibs, etc. Pickup is usually monthly, but pickup schedules are flexible.

PART II:
MARKETING THE PRACTICE

Chapter 8
Getting the Word Out

One of the most important parts of your dental practice, which is almost never discussed in school, is all about marketing and your practice website.

Marketing is going to be an enormous and ongoing project throughout your career. This part of the practice is very similar to learning new techniques in dentistry; think of it as continuing education, since it's evolving at a rapid rate in this digital age.

The absolute best marketing tool is word-of-mouth. If a patient comes in and tells you that you placed veneers on their friend and they want them as well, guess what? This patient is already sold! More than likely, they asked their friend how much the treatment had cost, which is helpful to you; cost is one of the biggest roadblocks for patients to accept treatment. These patients know roughly what similar treatment costs before they see you. These are the best patients to treat, in that you only have to concentrate on explaining the procedure and not on "selling" them on it.

Literature

There are marketing companies to fit every imaginable need, so sorting through them will take time and sometimes money. Whether you are a specialist or general dentist, your first step must be putting your name or practice name on different forms of literature. I recommend starting with a local printing company and begin by fabricating such items as: business cards, business card magnets, letterhead, hygiene bags, referral cards or pads with a clear map of the office location, etc.

Designing a logo is nice but is not a necessity at first. If you do decide you want one, put a call out on iFreelance.com for your logo, and spend possibly less than $250, but not more $500. Within 1-2 business days you will have dozens of artists' styles to choose from and can pick someone you feel you can work with comfortably.

Marketing You
Specialists should meet with as many dentists and their staff members as possible in their area, to introduce themselves and begin building the relationship. Ask what their treatment philosophies are and what their "ideal specialist" should do to treat their patient. I had numerous responses such as, "When we refer to a periodontist, we never see the patient again," and,

"Sometimes patients show up to our office with implants already placed, without consulting with me first." After hearing these answers, I made it a point to have excellent communication with the referring dentist before, during, and after treatment. Having a computerized office makes this task much easier. The resulting repeat referrals mean it was the right choice.

If you are going to practice as a general dentist, it's still a good idea to get out and meet your colleagues. Tell them that you are hungry for any extra work that they can throw your way. You will be surprised how many dentists don't remove teeth, or perform molar endo or other standard tasks. Make sure you drop off business cards and referral pads to make it easy to find your office.

Websites
Websites are another great way to promote your practice and inform your patients. With so much competition in the website arena, purchasing a site for less than $1,000 is very possible. The site can be hosted on GoDaddy.com for a few dollars a month.

Once you decide your domain name, search at the GoDaddy site to see if the domain is available. If so, follow the steps and sign up for around $12/year.

Your website designer will need the information after you sign up to be able to go in and make future changes to the site. Getting all the information and design is very time-consuming initially but it's well worth the additional growth to your business.

For my website, I made several Word documents on various topics. I also contacted other dentists to obtain their permission to use some of their materials on my site as well. I try to use my own cases whenever possible. During my residency, my program director made us take multiple before-and-after photos, and this is what I used on my own site.

A great way to get started developing your site is to search and find 8-10 sites with designs you like. Contact those doctors directly to see what content you can use. This will help the website design company and save you money in development time and effort, too.

SEO and Keywords
Many patients will search for a new dentist via the Internet. I very rarely look in the Yellow Pages for businesses; like most people, I use Google either on my phone or computer. Getting ranked high on the Google search list is just as important as the website, since what's the use of having a website if nobody can find you?

The person or company that designs your site should be able to help get the site listed in the top ten local searches. This is called SEO, or Search Engine Optimization, and it means making your site as easy to find as possible. One of the strongest ways to do this is using "keywords." For instance, the word "veneer" could be used as a keyword. When a potential patient searches for the word "veneer" plus the name of the town where you are practicing, this keyword, linked to your website, should drive the site higher on the Google list, versus a site that does not use the particular keyword.

Your web developer should be able to get a great site together for you in 2-4 weeks once they start. If you need something more complex, consider waiting and seeing how a simple 4-6 page site does to build your business, along with some great SEO for local searches.

Social Media

As you know by now, social media is HUGE! Sites such as Facebook and Twitter have millions of users and guess what? Your patients use these sites, too. Have your website designer design a Facebook page for your office. This is a great way to let your patients know about new products or services you are offering, or updates on what is new in dentistry. Offer patients a small coupon (egg., $5-10 off of their next cleaning) when they "Like" your page – they are endorsing your services, and by Liking it, it shows up on their pages and to their friends as well. Free advertising for you!

Newsletters

I sent out a monthly patient newsletter in 2011 for three months with little to no response or feedback. The newsletter was from a "cookie cutter" company that basically wrote generic articles and asked me to provide at least one article a month. The majority of the articles had to do with either a procedure we performed in the office or something to do with health and periodontal disease.

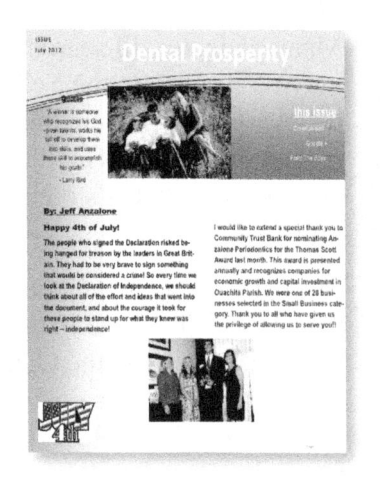

I stopped the newsletter and recently hired a wonderful marketing consultant who recommended restarting the newsletter, but this time, sharing information about my family and the practice as well as about me.

I was hesitant at first, wondering why anyone would want to know things about my family and me? Boy, was I wrong!! There is not a day that goes by that someone doesn't comment on the newsletter.

The original goal of hiring the marketing consultant was to increase new referrals from existing patients. The first two newsletters were a huge hit, and we have already received more new patients this month than we had received the previous six months! I guess people just want to know about other people! Why do you think Facebook is so popular?

Now I strongly recommend a monthly patient newsletter. This can be easily created using software that is probably already installed on your computer, like Microsoft Publisher. Or you can hire someone to do the design work on iFreelance.com or a similar site (guru.com, eLance.com, etc.) so long as you remember to create your own personal content.

As a dental specialist, I also send out regular newsletters to all my referring dentists. It's a great reminder to them of my existence, and it features useful information that continue to reinforce my value as a specialist.

Below is an example of a recent newsletter. Notice that I use exactly the same format and layout, and in some cases, the same content! Also note that it's tailored to the community, and imparts some really useful info — this particular issue is giving doctors new info about Google Plus and suggesting that they use this valuable marketing tool; it's not directly about dentistry, yet it's a powerful reminder of why they want to be in business as my partner.

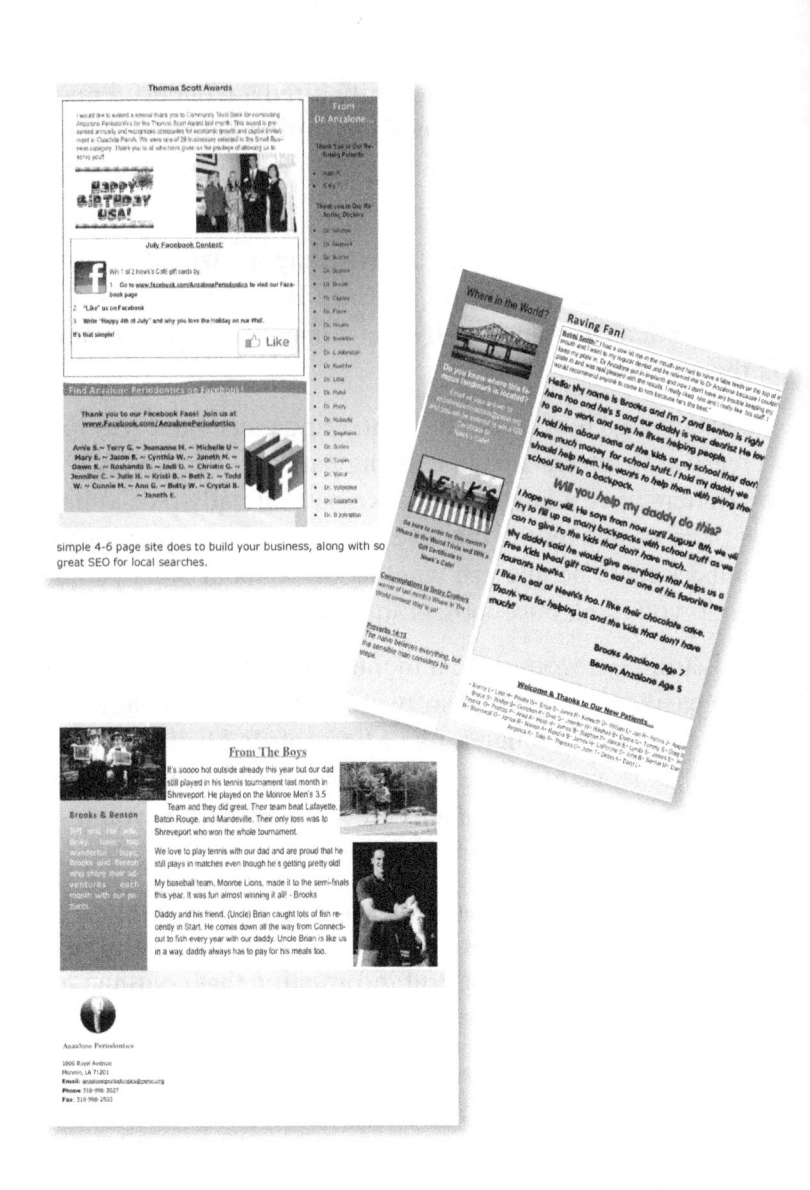

Page 4, the last page of BOTH newsletters, is identical. If you'd like help marketing your practice, I do consulting work for select clients only. For more information, please fax our office at **(318) 998-2503**.

Chapter 9
It's All About the Patients...Right?

Several years ago, a friend of mine, Robert Skrob, encouraged me to do something he had done some 10+ years ago that completely transformed his consulting business. Robert found out I was going to be in Orlando for a marketing meeting and encouraged me to go "undercover" at Disney. To be more specific, he told me to go through Disney's entire job interview process. At first I thought he was joking but came to find out he was as serious as a heart attack. Robert told me that what he had learned about attracting, hiring, training, and retaining employees was priceless. The kicker was he also had stumbled on to the secrets that Disney uses to instill its "Do whatever it takes to make the guest happy" culture.

Being the Disney enthusiast I am, there was no way I could pass up this opportunity. After my face-to-face interview, I was overwhelmed, not only by what I had learned but also because there was so much more to continue to learn. So, I did some research. I put all of this information together in a program (www.dentalpracticemagic.com) and now travel around the country presenting what I have learned to dentists and dental specialists.

Among the numerous things learned was how all Disney employees put their guests on a pedestal. The interview process took place in a building called the "Casting Center." Disney employees are not called employees; they are cast members. When someone goes to interview for a job at Disney, it's only fitting that he or she is going to "audition for a role" at the Casting Center.

Upon entering the building, the first thing I saw was 12 pillars arranged in a circle with the main Disney characters on top (see photo). Disney smartly portrays to potential cast members who is the most important to them. No matter who stands in the middle of that room, whether it is a janitor or the CEO, everyone has to look up to their main revenue source: the Disney characters.

I thought this was a cool idea, and so I want to pose a question to you: Do you and your staff focus on the main revenue source at your practice? Sometimes we can go off on a tangent and prejudge patients by what they are wearing, how they talk, what they look like, etc., instead of treating each patient like gold. Just because a patient comes to your office complaining of a single toothache doesn't mean that this person doesn't have several other teeth that need to be treated. And how about the potential for future referrals?

Make it a point to think of ways to place a specific and meaningful object in a common room shared by your team in your office that reminds everyone who they should be focusing on at all times ... your patients.

Remember, in every exceptionally *successful* dental practice, the patient is, is perceived as, and is *treated* as the most important asset.

Are You Attracting the Right Kind of Patients?
Now that we are on the subject of patients, let's talk more about something that is extremely important yet overlooked in dental school: how to attract the ideal patients we want to work with.

Dental schools across the country fall short on this huge aspect of a successful dental practice. We are trained solely to be clinically focused. Literally all continuing education meetings, seminars, and workshops teach us how to do things more efficiently, and they focus on new technology, the newest techniques, and the latest and greatest "hot" dental materials. Do you think purchasing a new 3D cone beam is going to get new patients to beat down your door? What about advertising to the general public that you own a laser? Things like a 3D cone beam and a new laser are great, but if you don't attract the right types of patients continuously, then you will go bankrupt. Trust me, there are thousands of dentists who do each year.

A Million-Dollar Lesson From Dan Kennedy

If you read the Introduction (please tell me you did), I mentioned that I was lucky enough to have been chosen as a finalist for Marketer of the Year at the Glazer-Kennedy SuperConference, one of the largest marketing conferences in the country. After wasting tens of thousands of dollars on marketing consultants, and advisors early in my career, I took matters into my own hands and began studying everything I could from the legendary marketing guru Dan Kennedy. I've read just about every book he has published and actually got my hands on one of his original home study courses, Magnetic Marketing. Magnetic Marketing is what sparked my interest in the world of direct marketing and lead generation (more on these topics later).

Magnetic Marketing consists of a study guide and cassette tapes (yes, tapes). I had to buy a cassette player since I had long since trashed all of mine. Long story short, I took one marketing campaign that was used by a restaurant, applied it to my practice, and voila! I actually got positive results, and I didn't need an advisor or a consultant to tell me what to do! After spending all of about $600 on printing, supplies, and postage, our first marketing campaign mailed out to existing patients that had unscheduled treatment netted over $18,000! How about that for a first-timer! Needless to say, I was hooked. Thanks, Dan!

One of Dan's first books, The Ultimate Marketing Plan, is chock-full of ideas that I used early on to establish and market my practice as the authority or go-to practice in my area. If you don't read any other marketing book out there, please read this one.

What's Your USP?
Do you have a USP or Unique Selling Proposition? Most dentists don't have a clue what I mean when I ask them this question. Your USP is simply why you exist as a practice/business. Basically, why should someone choose your practice over another one down the street? This is the basis for developing a solid marketing plan for your practice.

You must know the facts, features, benefits, and promises that your practice makes—inside out, backward, forward, and sideways. If you can't clearly articulate what makes your practice unique, how can you expect anyone else to care?

Finding your practice's USP is a job your entire team can contribute to. Make one of your team meetings focus solely on coming up with why prospective patients do business with you. One way of finding out is asking your current patients why they chose to come to you. You may hear things such as *"You guys have the best customer service I've ever experienced at a dental office"* or *"Dr. X is the only dentist who was able to completely erase my extreme dental phobia."*

Focus on the main pain points in dentistry (long wait, physical pain, expense), and set out to create your USP from solving one or several of these common problems.

One of the most famous USPs comes from the restaurant industry. I bet you can guess which company says this: "Fresh, hot pizza delivered in 30 minutes or less, guaranteed." Domino's used a major pain point (kids are starving when mom and dad get home from work). They knew that hardworking parents get home late and are usually too tired to cook. What better pain point to solve?! This simple USP made Domino's a billion-dollar company.

The Real Reason You Must Have a USP
Let's do a quick exercise. You can open up a copy of your local

Yellow Pages or use the internet. Search for dentists in your area and what do you find? That's right, your competition is literally all around (top, bottom, right, left) your advertisement. In both places, Yellow Pages and internet, you are literally surrounded by competing dental practices.

Roughly 10 to 15 years ago, the average person's attention span was about 15 minutes. Do you have any idea what it is now? Eight seconds. That's right. People have the attention span of a mosquito. What this means is that after eight seconds, if your message doesn't "attract" a prospective patient's attention— poof!—that prospect is gone, never to return.

So, both in the Yellow Pages and on the internet, you are presenting your practice information to the same prospective patient simultaneously with all of your competition. Survival of the fittest and the strongest will prevail.

Let's return to our little exercise. What do you notice about all of your competitor's messages? You know it. Everybody is saying the same thing. Here are a few examples I'm looking at right now in my local Yellow Pages:

- We cater to cowards
- Family Dentistry
- Cosmetic Dentistry
- Dentistry while you sleep
- We treat the whole family

Basically the list could go on and on. Trying to be everything to everyone is a bad mistake. Unfortunately, when we begin practicing, we imitate what everyone else is doing. I know I did.

Today, more than ever, we can no longer afford to be seen as *just another dentist*. Large corporate dental chains are metastasizing in the United States at an alarming rate. You must have a differential in place, and the way to start is by developing your practice's USP.

Stop Wasting Money!
The next time you are getting ready to submit an ad for a local newspaper, high school sports program, or magazine—or you're asked to renew your Yellow Pages ad—please stop and reread what I'm getting ready to tell you. There's nothing that churns my stomach more than to flip through local newspapers, magazines, etc., and see all types of businesses and companies wasting their hard-earned dollars on ineffective and basically dumb marketing.

Let's take a look at the example below to see what I mean:

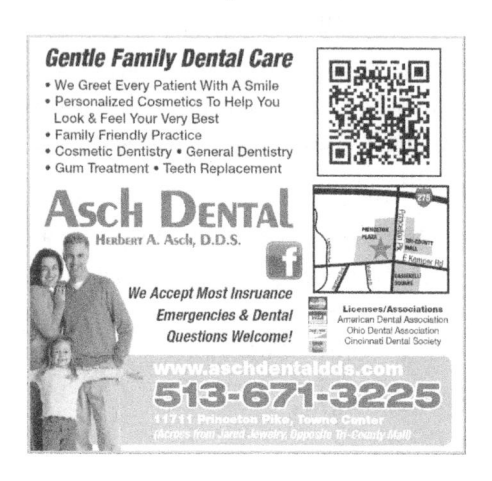

Gentle Family Dental Care
- We Greet Every Patient With A Smile
- Personalized Cosmetics To Help You Look & Feel Your Very Best
- Family Friendly Practice
- Cosmetic Dentistry • General Dentistry
- Gum Treatment • Teeth Replacement

Asch Dental
Herbert A. Asch, D.D.S.

We Accept Most Insruance
Emergencies & Dental
Questions Welcome!

Licenses/Associations
American Dental Association
Ohio Dental Association
Cincinnati Dental Society

www.aschdentaldds.com
513-671-3225
11711 Princeton Pike, Towne Center
(Across from Jared Jewelry, Opposite Tri-County Mall)

Would you agree that this is a typical ad that you might find in your local Yellow Pages, newspaper, or magazine? I would be willing to wager that this is what the majority of your competitors' advertisements look like. Most advertising salespeople ask for a business card and simply create an ad from it—an ad that doesn't attract new patients.

I could write an entire book on how to create effective dental advertising to maintain a steady stream of patients, but an overview here will have to suffice.

Rule #1: Create a Catchy Headline

First, you must have an eye-catching headline. **"Gentle Family Dental Care"** is by no means original and definitely doesn't stand out to catch your eye (remember, you have eight seconds). So, here is Rule #1: Create a unique and catchy headline that attracts the types of patients you want to treat.

An example of an attention-grabbing headline would be something like **"Do You Hate Going to the Dentist?"** This headline could lead into an advertisement regarding sedation dentistry. How about this one: **"Are You Embarrassed to Smile in Public?"** This could lead into a cosmetic advertisement. Your headline should create an awareness of a need or a desire. Be creative. Questions make the best headlines.

Now that you have grabbed a prospective patient's attention, listing all of your services or explaining that you accept most dental insurances is a sure way to lose this person.

Rule #2: Add Some Drama

Your ad's content must be relevant to the headline and add drama. No, I'm not talking about dental office drama, but drama that will make you seem intriguing and less boring than all the other dentists. Simply using before and after pictures or, better yet, patient testimonials with pictures is highly effective.

Here's an example of one our practice's testimonials:

Patient X: "I was referred to Anzalone Periodontics to replace some teeth with dental implants. My main concerns were pain during/after the procedure and time off work. My expectations were explained and met, the staff was very nice, and Dr. Anzalone also called the evening after the procedure to check on me."

Rule #3: Make Them an Offer

The next thing to put in your advertisement is a <u>specific</u> <u>offer</u>. This is something you give to potential patients in return for their contact information. It could be to call for a Free Consultation or to go to a website to download a Free Report or eBook. No matter what you choose to offer, choose something.

FREE OFFER!
After writing about the correct way to advertise, I feel compelled to give you, the reader, a special offer. If you have any type of advertisement that you are getting ready to run (or are currently running) and would like me to critique it for FREE, fax it to 318.998.2503.

In the subject line, write: <u>Free Ad Critique</u> followed by the title of this book.

Each purchaser of this book will receive one Free Critique—unless I'm so overwhelmed by the response that I have to rethink my offer. This offer may expire at any time.

In the example advertisement above, did you notice anything being offered in return for a prospective patient's contact information? Think through what you want your prospective patients to do—and ask them to do it.

Rule #4: Create a Sense of Urgency With a Deadline

The majority of the general public, including myself, procrastinates with a capital "P." If we have a project due, we tend to wait until the last minute to start on it, right? Packing for vacation usually starts the night before or, for some, the morning of the trip. Yikes!

Automobile and furniture dealers tend to get this right by running 48 or 72 hour only sales. This creates a sense of urgency and gives a hard deadline to respond by.

Example: "This Weekend Only: 40% Off All Leather Chairs!"

Advertisements for our practice usually set a deadline for roughly two weeks after an ad runs. Make sure your staff members are given some type of advance notice so they can prepare for the influx of calls!

Rule #5: Scarcity Rules
If you are running a new patient special or are giving away a free electric toothbrush, consider limiting the number of supplies, at least on paper. Supply and demand works like a charm when presenting your offer.

The first time we ran a promotion to current patients offering a discount for unscheduled treatment, we also offered a free Sonicare toothbrush to the first 13 callers. We actually had some patients call just to get the free toothbrush, wanting to know if they were one of the first 13 callers! If we hadn't limited our offer, our patients wouldn't have had this sense of urgency to call right away.

Following these simple rules every single time you run an advertisement will generate thousands of dollars. It does for me.

Chapter 10
No-Resistance Selling
Getting a Yes! for Treatment

Let's take a trip down memory lane. For some of us, this trip is going to be longer than for others. Let's return to the days when we were dental students, specifically when we were learning how to talk to patients about the treatments they needed. During some type of treatment planning or oral diagnosis course, we received hands-on training with patients. Our teachers instructed us to evaluate a patient's radiographs, perform a full examination, list every type of restoration needed, and then explain the treatments to our patient over the next two hours.

We were taught to explain each restoration or recommended treatment in detail so that the patient fully understood what needed to be done. If you were to go back and put yourself in your patients' shoes, you would realize that most of them were fully convinced that the treatment would either be free or extremely low in price since you were still a student. That's why they had come to a dental school for their treatment in the first place.

So, what did we learn? All we had to do to get our patients to accept treatment was what? Make a list, check it twice, find out who's naughty or nice? Not exactly. Yes, we did list out all the treatment that our dental school patients needed, but that is not why they accepted treatment. The only thing they wanted while they were there was to get their teeth fixed dirt cheap. That's it. Why else would someone subject themselves to a three- or four-hour appointment for a single molar root canal? But when we left dental school, we fully believed that all we had to do to get a patient to accept treatment was to explain each procedure in detail. Do you still think that is what patients really want?

Out of everything that dental schools across the country fall short on teaching dentists, I believe that the lack of education regarding how to build a relationship with patients, get them to accept treatment, obtain referrals, and get patients to come back for future treatment is the greatest disservice to future dentists.

Once you master the entire new patient process from start to finish, you should see amazing results duplicated month after month. All of the incremental steps we are going to discuss will help build on each other to get your patients to do business with you. People want to do business with people they know, like, and trust. I know I do.

I'm in the process of writing an entire book about building trust-based relationships with patients, but I'll go ahead and give you the "CliffsNotes" version of it now.

Are You Scaring Away Your Patients?

How many times have you walked into a place of business and after the salesman asks if he can help you, you give him the ole "I'm just looking" line? I'm sure plenty. Why do we do this? We do this because we don't like being sold to. In a nutshell, we don't like or trust salespeople.

What happens when someone dressed in a suit and tie knocks on your front door on a Saturday morning? If you have kids like I do, you tell them not to answer that door and to hide behind the curtains until the guy is gone, right? Disdain for salespeople is usually ingrained in us from some type of childhood experience we have had with our parents, teachers, or other influential adults.

If you or your staff members are coming across as salespeople, you will surely drive folks out of your practice.

Case Acceptance

Howard Farran, CEO of Dentaltown, wrote an article in 2014 regarding case acceptance. He stated that the average general practice in the United States has a 30 to 35 percent case acceptance rate.

Let's assume that each one of the new patients that comes through your door is initially worth $1,000. If your practice fits in with the national average of case acceptance, you are losing $6,000 to $7,000 for every 10 new patients you see. That's a lot of dough.

Do you track your case acceptance? Most dentists don't. You can't manage what you don't measure. Successful sports teams track and measure every statistic imaginable. That's one of the reasons they perform so well. They focus on the problem areas and then practice resolving them.

I've made it my mission to educate as many dentists as possible about the number of patients who are leaving their practices each week without a return appointment. The amount of lost revenue is alarming.

It's for this reason that I have put together an entire *New Patient Case Acceptance System* (www.caseacceptancesystem.com) that teaches everything from A to Z about becoming a respected, authoritative, expert practice and how to leverage your expertise to attract quality patients who are ready to begin treatment.

The remainder of this chapter will give give you an overview of ways to beat the national case acceptance average of 30 to 35 percent.

The Initial Call
One of the best decisions I made years ago was to train my staff on the proper way to answer the phone to achieve the goal of scheduling new patient visits. I'm in no way affiliated with the *Scheduling Institute* but do highly recommend this organization or one like it to train your team.

I first heard the Scheduling Institute's owner, Jay Geier, speak during a small meeting of periodontists in New Orleans. It was in the early years when Jay still did small group events. I had no idea who he was or what he was about at the time. One of the first things he did was take out a New Orleans phonebook and place a call to a randomly selected local dental office. He played the part of a prospective patient and put the call on speaker so that everyone in the room could hear. I was flabbergasted by what I heard. The call was finally answered after about 9 or 10 rings. The receptionist's rude and annoyed attitude was apparent. She answered Jay's questions with sighing and no patience whatsoever. Needless to say, no appointment was given or contact information captured. This was eye opening. Like the other dentists in the area, I assumed that my team knew how to answer the phone properly and appoint patients. But did they? How would I know if I had never checked?

During a break, the meeting attendees began talking amongst themselves. One of my colleagues told me there was NO WAY that what we had just heard was going on in his office. We decided to put his belief to the test. With my phone on speaker, I dialed his office.

I began the call by saying I was new to town and needed a dental implant. I asked the receptionist if the practice took a particular dental insurance. She instructed me to call the number on the back of my insurance card with a list of dental codes she provided and then abruptly hung up. The ashen look on my friend's face said it all!

Needless to say, we both signed up our offices to have Jay's team train us on answering the phone, and the results have been exceptional. This is something that must be continually monitored, and I now monitor, record, and track every inbound call.

If you have never had someone mystery shop your practice, put this book down and arrange for someone to do it ASAP.

Warning: Be prepared to be sick to your stomach when you listen to the calls.

But let me follow up my warning with some encouragement. When you uncover poor phone customer service at your office, don't think of it as a bad thing; think of it this way. You have a problem, the problem has never been addressed before, and now you know there are solutions to this specific problem. Let's face it. Ultimately all of the problems in our office come back to us, the doctor. It was my fault that I hadn't trained my staff properly on answering the phone. Once I began monitoring inbound calls, I was able to manage this important aspect of my practice.

Not Having a Differential
Do you remember when we discussed forming your USP? Your USP is why patients should choose you over someone else to take care of their dental needs. It's your way of showing how you and your practice are different. You must have a differential. By differential, I don't mean touting that you are the lowest priced dentist in town. A strong pricing strategy has everything to do with your positioning and your marketplace differential. Strong positioning allows you to attract patients who want the best results and are willing to pay for it. And it eliminates having to deal with patients you *don't* want to work with.

Likewise, having a weak, or even worse, *no* differential, puts you at the mercy of your patients. Since you're offering them nothing different from anyone else, they perceive you as being average (at best), and that's why you start getting price resistance and uncertainty when it comes to case acceptance.

Not Knowing What Your Patients Really Want
My good friend Fred Joyal, co-founder of 1-800-DENTIST, told me during one of our monthly marketing calls that the #1 thing a patient is seeking from a dentist is to be made to feel important. That's it. They don't want to be just another number.

Patients want you to have a good bedside manner, and they want to feel safe—especially if you're performing a surgery or a complicated procedure. They want to feel like they can trust you.

I'm going to let you in on a little secret you definitely *don't* know: You want to let your patients know that you have a good bedside manner, that you are skilled, and that they can trust you and feel safe with you **BEFORE they come into your office, not *after* they have already arrived.**

When patients arrive at a dental office, they are likely to be feeling defensive and anxious, and many are experiencing physical pain or discomfort. As a result, they will *not* be very open to hearing or processing much of what you might say or do—even if it's for their own benefit.

When you give your patients what they want *prior* to their visit, instead of feeling anxious when they come into your office, they will feel safe. This is because **they feel like they already know you.** And when someone feels like they know you, they're far more open to any kind of treatment recommendations you might make.

Which causes case acceptance to go up, *dramatically* ... Does this make sense? Good. Oh, and by the way, there are a few *other* things virtually all patients want as well. And again, they should know you possess each one of these qualities before they arrive at your office:

1. **Enthusiasm - They want to know you're excited about what you do.** Because if you're not excited about it, why should they be?
2. **Believability - Should they believe you when you make a suggestion?** Or is there a chance that your recommendations are more important to you (based on financial gain) and less important to their oral health? This is where your use of testimonials from

other patients helps you out. After all, what others say about you is far more important than whatever you have to say about yourself.
3. **Credibility - Are you qualified to be working on their specific problem, and are your recommendations based on experience or on a "hunch" about things?** Credibility issues are best resolved by sharing before and after photos, comments from other patients, and case studies of specific problems you've solved for specific patients.
4. **Competence and skill level - Have you had special training?** If so, make sure you've communicated this to your patients *ahead* of time. Especially if this training is relevant to the particular dental problems they're coming to see you about.

At this point you're probably thinking, "Yes, this sounds really smart. But how on earth can you communicate all these things in one fell swoop, and how do you do all this before you meet with your patient?" Let me let you in on a little secret about how I stumbled onto all of this ...

How Disney Can Help Our Case Acceptance Rates

Have you been to a Disney property? Out of all the companies and businesses out there, Disney is my number one go-to source for practice-building information. Vacationing at Disney is the least likely thing you might think of doing when you want to come up with a great practice-building idea, right? Well, I got one of my practice's most effective and profitable ideas while riding on Disney's bus system, the Magical Express.

If you've been to Disney World and stayed at a Disney property, you've more than likely experienced the Magical Express. This transportation service shuttles guests to and from the Orlando airport. There's no stopping for food or souvenirs while on board. Disney wants you to go from the airport straight to the theme park. They know once you're there, you are trapped into purchasing everything (food, snacks, merchandise, etc.) behind Disney's gates.

Several years ago, while riding on the Magical Express to my resort, I started noticing something unique about the onboard TV monitors. Early on in my Disney-going experiences, cartoons played the majority of the time, but Disney keeps getting smarter and smarter. Over time, I noticed a change.

Today, cartoons make up a small portion of air time, and the remainder is all about providing guests information about their destination. The choice of information has been gleaned by surveying guests about what they need to know before getting to a park. Now guests can learn about the different shows being offered (e.g., Cirque du Soleil), merchandise that can be purchased and delivered to the guest room, the Disney Vacation Club (Disney's form of timeshare properties), and most important, what to expect when you arrive.

Disney can be an overwhelming place the first time you visit. The people at Disney know this so they explain the main concerns guests might have such as the check-in process at the resort. The video covers how luggage
is handled and sent to your room, where the check-in desks are located, and how to use your room key (which is now a "Magic Band" worn on your wrist).

If you treat baby boomers in your practice (which is the largest and fastest growing segment of the population), you should know what Disney knows. Baby boomers do NOT like surprises. This is one of the reasons why Disney provides helpful information to guests before they arrive at the parks or one of the Disney hotels.

Other companies such as Audi and Eleven James also send their customers information to pre-meet them, which helps begin the relationship process. After studying how Disney and other companies prepare their customers to have a good experience, I asked myself the question "How can I apply this to my practice?" I wanted to find a way to get important information into the hands of my new patients BEFORE they arrived at our office.

What do most dentists do when a new patient calls and, we hope, is appointed? Most do nothing. A handful might send some type of welcome letter, or perhaps a few office forms to be filled out before the visit, but that's about it.

Instead, picture your patients receiving a large box in the mail (part of the New Patient Case Acceptance System) before their appointment with you. This box is stuffed with frequently asked questions, proof, testimonials, books, booklets, DVDs, CDs, literally mind-blowing stuff! I guarantee you they will have never experienced anything like this from any other dentist. Talk about having a differential!

Now, I want to take this differential a step further and discuss with you the value of writing a book. Before you start telling yourself that you don't know how or have time to author a book, let me tell you about my experiences in the next chapter.

Chapter 11:
How to Become THE Authority Dental Practice in Your Town

How many dentists in your area are authors? I'd be willing to bet zero, nada, zilch. As an author, you will be seen in a different light. There is no more essential tool of authority than authorship. Heck, what do the first six letters of "authority" spell anyway? That's right, author.

In his fantastic book *Influence: The Psychology of Persuasion*, Dr. Robert Cialdini discusses six key principles of influence to ethically persuade others. One of these six principles is <u>authority</u>. He states that when people desire to obtain information about a certain topic or subject, they universally seek out credible, trustworthy sources of authority to tell them what they should be doing. One of the top sources of this information will come from those who have written books about the subject of interest.

I am not recommending that you write a book to make millions of dollars by selling it in bookstores (which would be nice). I recommend using your book for <u>direct distribution</u> to prospective and new patients instead of other common marketing materials such as business cards and brochures. Remember our discussion regarding the public's general dislike of salespeople? Salesmen have brochures; trusted authority experts have books. Enough said.

How to Lower Price Sensitivity

For most dental practices, the quality patient is a reader. Nowadays, with people constantly connected to their phones and tablets, it's becoming more and more important to target specific niches for our practices.

If someone has a question about something pertaining to dentistry, say dental implants, many will "Google" the term, post a question to their friends on Facebook, or search online forums. It's amazing the amount of free content that is available 24/7.

In contrast, consider a prospective patient who wants to know more about how dental implants can help her and instead searches Amazon for credible authors. Better yet, she drives to a local bookstore and actually spends money on books before returning home to read in the comfort of her own home. This individual will be less price sensitive than the "shopper" patient who calls your office and asks, "What do you charge for dental implants?"

After years of using different media, including books, to market my practice, I can attest that patients who invested time in reading my books were more committed to buying and less likely to comparison shop.

Here's one example of how leveraging a book can improve advertising results. In a study of medical clinic advertising, ads that offered a free consultation were compared to ads that also offered the free consult but added a free book. Almost 80 percent of the prospective patients who arrived to their appointment via the book offer accepted the recommended treatment versus 50 percent of those who responded to the free consult only ad. Plus, the average six-month dollar value of the book-offer patients was nearly double that of non-book patients. Not a bad response by simply adding a book to the marketing mix.

How to Market to Prospective Patients Without Really Marketing

The general public is inundated with thousands upon thousands of marketing and advertising messages daily. Think about every marketing message you have encountered today. You may have noticed a sign on the side of a bus, listened to radio ads on your way to work, noticed them on the side of your coffee cup, watched TV or website ads, or glanced over numerous ones while reading the morning paper. Most people become so annoyed by the constant bombardment of advertisements that they begin automatically to try to avoid them at all costs.

I don't know about you, but if I'm watching a television program, I typically use the time when commercials are airing to get a snack or take a bathroom break. If I'm listening to the radio in my truck, I click to a new station when ads start playing.

Don't get me wrong. Effective ads are floating around out there, but with the constant barrage coming at us from all different media, advertisements have to have something unique or eye-catching to grab our attention. If they don't, people do whatever they can to avoid them. And if you're the one doing such advertising, people are avoiding your practice.

You can sidestep this problem by using a book in your marketing. Our patients love receiving our books and routinely share them with others, resulting in increased patient to patient referrals. Our patients don't view our books as an advertisement, but rather as a helpful source of dental information.

Your goal is to make prospective patients focus totally on your message only. By using the strategies in this chapter, you have a great opportunity to do this.

Here's something else that dental school lacked when it came to educating us ... lead generation.

Generating Leads With Your Book
If there is one thing dental school SHOULD have educated us about, it is how to get prospective patients who are somewhat interested in our services to "raise their hand" to get more information. This, in a nutshell, is lead generation. A lead is an individual who is searching for information or a provider to help with his or her problem.

The original idea to write a book for our patients came from an unlikely source, a Beverly Hills cosmetic surgeon, Dr. Bob Kotler. Unlike most health care providers, Dr. Kotler smartly shifted all of his marketing efforts to focus on his book instead of his services. As you can imagine, there's probably a plastic surgeon on every corner of Beverly Hills. By advertising a book rather than his practice, the good doctor immediately stood out, thus providing a differential.

Websites

Humor me for a second. Locate a computer near you and do a quick search for dentists in your area. For example, go to Google and put in your town's name and the word "dentist." I hope you see your website on the first page of the search results! Now, I want you to browse around some of your competitor's websites. I'm actually looking at one now. What do you see at the top of all of these websites? Let me guess: the practice name, a logo, and a large picture of a smiling person imitating a patient.

After researching thousands of websites, I have noticed a recurring trend. Over 90 percent of dental websites use the top third of their homepage as nothing more than an announcement of the practice name and logo. Unfortunately, they are wasting this space. The top third of the homepage is the most IMPORTANT part of the site!

The #1 reason why your website exists is NOT to educate but to capture. Capture what? You guessed it, capture leads via lead generation. There is no better way to do this than by giving something for free ... such as a book.

I'm sure there have been times when you have visited a website and have been asked for contact information in exchange for a free report or book. You can do the same thing! When you use your book as a lead generation method, you will know who has visited your website. You want to attract patients who are really interested in your services, and your book will "flush" them out, so to speak. What's the point of having a website if you have no idea how many prospects are browsing it and have no way to get in touch with them?

Here's a screen shot of our homepage:

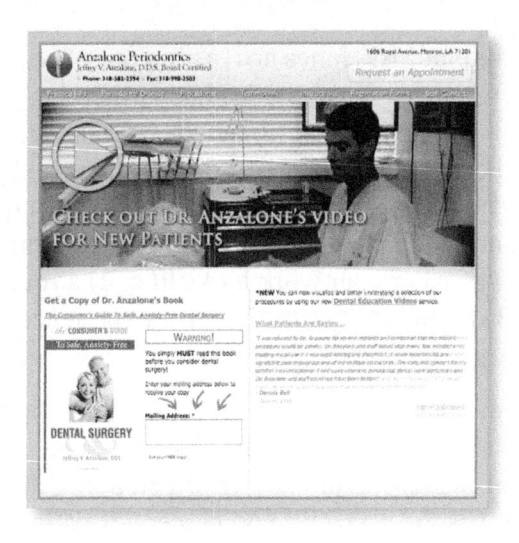

I have dedicated the entire homepage to generating leads (book opt-in), beginning the relationship process (office tour video at the top), and making it easy for the handful of patients who want to schedule an appointment as soon as possible (Request an Appointment button).

If you have a website, take a long, hard look at the first page a prospective patient encounters. Do you have a way to obtain contact information for future follow-up? If not, have your webmaster create something for you.

Using a Book as the Ultimate Referral Tool
One of the top sources for new patients in your practice will always be the ones who arrive as referrals via current or former patients. Several things differentiate a "word of mouth" referral

from a patient who arrives in your office after seeing your name or advertisement elsewhere. Referred patients are much less price sensitive. They usually have an idea of the type of dentistry they want as well as a ballpark figure of what it will cost. (The patients who referred them probably had the same type of treatment and shared the cost with them.)

Here's an example: Mrs. Jones arrives in your office via direct referral from Mrs. Sally, her bridge partner. Last month, you delivered four veneers on Mrs. Sally's front teeth, and she couldn't help showing them off during the weekly bridge match. Upon noticing your nice work, Mrs. Jones inquired about them and, voila, a new patient has headed your way with: 1) knowledge of what your work looks like; 2) a rough estimate of cost; and 3) knowledge of the positive experience Mrs. Jones had with you and your team.

Research shows that around 20 percent of your patients will freely send their friends and family. Usually 20 percent will not refer at all for one reason or another. If I'm doing the math correctly, that leaves the remaining 60 percent of patients who will more than likely refer—but only if you have a system in place to encourage them to do so.

Asking patients to refer you can be awkward. Using a book makes asking a patient for a referral much easier. Have you ever heard of the phrase "pass-along effect"? A book is an example of using a pass-along effect to bring a stream of referrals into the practice. Here's how this works:

You just finished delivering an all-ceramic crown on tooth #8 for Mrs. Smith. After you hand her a mirror to show off your handiwork, she excitedly states how much she loves the color and shape and that you did a fantastic job.

The absolute best time to ask a patient for a referral is after she has complimented you. In this case, Mrs. Smith has complimented you on your work, and now you are armed and ready to start the process of asking for a referral. So, you ask her if she would mind doing you a favor and wait for a reply. After she says that she would love to do something for you, it is an easy and natural thing to ask her to share your book with people she knows. Using a book as a referral tool is much easier than directly asking her to send over family or friends who may need your services.

Here is the main reason dental offices <u>don't</u> ask for patient to patient referrals. It can be awkward, or you may think it makes you sound desperate to ask. A book makes the transition to asking for referrals much smoother. We typically say something like, "Mrs. Smith, would you mind giving out copies of our book to folks you think could use our help?"

How easy is that?

Honestly, how much do your patients really know about the exact process of the work you perform on them? It is much easier for your patients to hand your book to someone who is missing a tooth and say, "Go see my dentist! He's a great guy, and he can fix your smile" than to explain what you actually do. This is what the pass-along effect is all about. You're passing along a source of information that your patients can pass along to others.

Most marketing consultants will have you hand out slick cards with your name on them, possibly with some type of free offer (exam, X-ray, etc.). Cards like these usually don't last long before they hit the trash can. But if you give someone a book, he is MUCH less likely to throw it away. There's something hard about throwing away a book (even if you don't read it).

There is no advertising medium you currently use or will use in the future where a book won't improve your results.

Chapter 12
The Rest of What They Didn't Teach You

Over the past several years, I have found some invaluable tips and lessons (some the hard way) that I am passing on to you. Some of these tips will save you money, others will save you time (and therefore money), and all will help ensure you have a thriving practice with repeat clients.

First Impressions
Your waiting room is the chance for you to make a great first impression, so make sure it's friendly and well-maintained. Dead plants, old magazines, dust, mis-matched furniture, bare white walls or cheap corporate art will all combine with the patient's natural misgivings about the procedure. If your waiting room is dingy, they may think your equipment is, too!

I recently purchased a TV and hung it in the waiting room to post things like: before-and-after pictures, welcome messages to new patients, our website, information about our Facebook Business Page, pictures of the staff, pictures of our family, selected education videos, and any contests or promotions we are offering. This is easily accomplished via our patient education video software (see Consult-Pro, below). The TV was connected to a computer with the software on it, and acts as an additional computer monitor.

You or someone you hire can make presentations and keep them updated regularly. Every day in my office a patient comments on either a video or picture that they saw on our waiting room television screen. Occasionally, patients tell me that they have no questions about their recommended treatment because the video in the waiting room explained it all. Talk about a huge consultation time saver!

Your patients are going to need something to read in the waiting room, and you don't want them to see the same old thing if they have to come in for multiple visits, plus it makes you look up-todate when your news is. A great magazine service to consider is Ebsco Magazines (www.ebscomags.com.) You can choose to subscribe to multiple magazines on this site and pay an annual fee. The price for each magazine subscription is considerably lower than the stand-alone price. Don't forget to consider ALL your patients when you order these; not just the ones you personally would like to read.

Testimonials
As early in your career as possible, begin taking before and after pictures. You may have some of these from your training; if so, put together a booklet showing patients what you can do for them. Place these booklets in the waiting room as it's a great practice builder and will boost your patient's confidence in you.

Also, store all of these pictures on a computer for possible future speaking engagements, powerpoint presentations, presentations to patients, newsletters, etc.

Making Patients Comfortable
You're the dentist; they're the patient. You think this stuff is cool; they're terrified and they may even hate the thought of having to see you. Don't take it personally. I never had a bad experience with my dentist, so it didn't occur to me that someone might not enjoy seeing me or being in my care. Today, I practice dental surgery, the majority of my patients are sedated when I see them, and they are happy not to remember a thing about their surgery afterwards.

It's your job to make your patients as comfortable as possible and that often means educating them. A lot of the pain is in their head, before any procedure takes place. Getting them wellprepared as well as educated will go a long way towards both relaxing them and giving you repeat business, since often dentists overlook this vital piece of marketing, their "bedside manner."

Consider purchasing patient education software such as Consult Pro or Caesy. I was frustrated trying to explain different procedures to patients and then began using Consult Pro. Their numerous education videos that can be shown or emailed to the patient, which makes explaining the procedure a snap. You can also insert before-and-after pictures into the presentations and print all material for the patient to take home. This software has gotten the point across better than I can, saved me time, and increased our case acceptance.

Continuing Education
Make sure you don't fall into the mindset of the majority of dentists upon graduating. I'm sure you have already heard it, "As soon as I graduate, I'm never going to study or take an exam again!" This is detrimental thinking and will do nothing for you or your practice. Get into the habit of constantly reading to better yourself as a person, leader (yes, you are a leader, so start thinking of yourself as one), clinician, mother/father, etc.

Especially ingest everything you can regarding marketing. Don't just focus on dental marketing; focus on what other businesses are doing that is working and apply it to your practice. Whether you are selling services or widgets, smart business habits are the same in any small growing business. It's amazing the marketing information you can learn and implement from other types of businesses.

A great monthly newsletter that has really helped me learn about and network with different businesses and consultants can be found at https://gkic.infusionsoft.com/go/newmifge/janzal. This newsletter has been a terrific asset to my practice.

My Final Piece of Advice
As you can see from the amount of information we covered in this book, setting up a dental practice is actually a complex operation where you have to think strategically, plan methodically, and execute smartly. Don't try to accomplish all these tasks while still in your last year of dental school. You have the rest of your life to practice so take it slow and as debt-free as possible.

Bonus Chapter

A good friend of mine, Dr. Brian Evans, trained with me at LSU in Periodontics. I asked him to share his story regarding his military training. For those of you who are looking for ways to pay for your dental career and don't want to acquire a huge student loan debt load, military service may be right for you. His story is below:

*The Military Avenue To Beginning
a Debt-Free Dental Career
by Dr. Brian Evans*

"You're going into the military?"

"What a waste of time!"

"They will own you and you can't make any money that way!"

"You'll be shipped overseas!"

Those are just a few of the examples I recall of conversations with my dental classmates on late nights after parties or during our breaks. Joining the military was looked down upon by many of my classmates, at least where I went to school, and while I didn't feel ridiculed, I certainly developed some insecurities once I signed the dotted line and stated my oath to defend our country.

I remember taking the oath so clearly. I arrived at the New Orleans Naval Base front gate in my civilian polo shirt and blue jeans and was met by a stoic MP. I didn't know whether to salute him or give him my papers. He gave me the ten different steps to get a vehicle pass and find my way on base, directing me to a small office in the recruiting department. When I finally found the office, reality truly set in: *I'm really doing this and I'm not so sure I want to.*

I grew up in a very modest household. My parents could not afford to pay for college, let alone grad school. I was fortunate to grow up playing golf, so I was able to get out of college with minimal debt because of academic and golf scholarships, and as much help as my parents could offer. My classmates told me military dentistry was all getting patients in and out to go to war and that ultimately, the payback for school loans was not worth it. They said I could easily make up for that in private practice in a couple of years. Besides, loan rates were so low, I could pay them off for the rest of my career without thinking much about them.

At the same time, military recruiters were telling me I would have the time of my life with opportunities to practice full-scope dentistry for half a day, while I spent the other half relaxing on a beach in Rota, Spain or Hawaii, all while the military paid me, with full medical benefits and dental specialty pay. I decided to fill out the paperwork.

The process to join the military was quite laborious. There were piles of paperwork to fill out and a medical examination I had to pass. I probably feared the medical exam more than any because of the horror stories I heard of having to turn and cough and what happened next, but it never did. In fact, the exam was fairly innocuous and I passed easily. I also applied for and received the Navy Health Professions Scholarship Program(HPSP) which would make me a commissioned officer with the rank of Ensign.

So on my way to take my oath, though I had thoughts of turning around and leaving, I also realized this was my opportunity to see the world and practice dentistry. The military would pay for my school loans, and I was going to take the chance on them, just as they were taking a chance on me.

Life was good that summer between first and second year of dental school.

I reaped the good part of my decision, and when it was time to pay tuition and buy books the next year, my Uncle Sam took care of me. I still remember the sense of satisfaction I felt knowing my loan tally would no longer be rising. I was also receiving a monthly stipend, so weekend life got a lot better. I reacquainted myself with the finer beers and bar food of New Orleans.

That same summer, I met my wife, Sue, who I've been married to now for ten years. The decision I had made to join the Navy, be a care-free, single man and see the world was suddenly complicated. My wife was in Tulane medical school, also between her first and second years. As we began to date, Sue introduced me to the wonderful restaurants New Orleans had to offer, laying the groundwork for my life as a future foodie.

She also made me realize our relationship, which was getting more serious, was going to be difficult to maintain with the uncertainty of where life would take us upon graduation. Sue would be matched in a residency somewhere and I would be subject to wherever the Navy stationed me among its numerous bases and ships throughout the world. Things started to look challenging and we both became fearful and depressed about having a future that didn't involve the other. Of course I proposed to Sue.

To make matters worse, I also developed an interest in periodontics in the beginning of my junior year and knew that going directly into a Periodontics residency was unlikely, given my Navy commitment immediately following dental school graduation.

Luckily, after researching my options and seeking out a periodontal resident at my school who was a former Navy periodontist, I found there was a way: I could apply and get into a periodontics residency, defer my Navy obligation until after residency, and also potentially match with my now-fiancée, all still keeping my debt accumulation for school at a stand still.

There was hope!

The Navy program I found was called NADDS, or Naval Active Duty for the Delay of Specialists program. In the NADDS program, you become interested in one of the dental specialties, get accepted into a program and apply for a deferment to complete the residency before you begin serving in the Navy. The student gets to continue training in an interest he or she has developed in dental school, and the Navy gets a specialist fresh out of training to help support the fleet. The key factor in receiving such deferment is based on the needs of the Navy Dental Corps. They convene a board of Naval Dental Officers (usually higher-ranking officers) who project the needs of the Navy.

For example, during my application process, which again was quite laborious, filled with paperwork and requiring good to excellent grades, the NADDS board concluded he Navy would need four periodontists the year I would complete my residency. This projection is based on how many periodontists the Navy would be expected to retire and how many Periodontal Billets would be available. Well, with a little luck, knowing a Captain on the board, and my good grades I was granted a deferment.

I was thrilled when I heard the news. I had taken a risk as I had applied to several periodontal programs (as my school was first choice) and was accepted in September, yet could not confirm I would be starting residency as the NADDS board did not come to a decision until December. Fortunately, my program director was gracious enough to hold the spot contingent upon my deferment.

The other part of the challenge was making sure Sue could match in a residency in the same city. It was really a wonderful day when we found out that she had, and we would be together.

The next three years were some of the toughest academically and clinically for both of us, as we were involved in our own intense dental and medical residencies. But we were together; we married the day before we both graduated from medical and dental school, and for at least the next three years did not have to worry about where life and the Navy would take us.

The NADDS program did offer me the option to continue to receive a stipend, and would have paid for my residency. After discussing it with my wife, I declined, as this would have incurred three more years of obligation on top of my current three-year commitment. That left my wife and me to fend for ourselves, paying for living expenses, my residency tuition and other bills.

We had Sue's small residency salary and I moonlighted to help out. Later, I did take out a couple of smaller loans to help cover tuition as the extra job and her residency salary didn't exactly make ends meet. The first year my wife and I were married, it was very tough. We were both stressed with residency and financially; Sue was the "spender" and I was the "tightwad." Our money styles didn't mix, and our marriage was threatened. It all came to a head with a few overwhelming bills. Thanks to Dr. Jeff, who introduced us to Dave Ramsey after our first year of residency, we were guided towards Financial Peace, we got on track and have never looked back.

With our residencies winding down, the big question was, where would the Navy be sending me? To complicate matters, Sue had developed an interest in another specialty and wanted to apply for another residency. In talking with the Naval Detailer, they ultimately decided to station me in Norfolk, VA, home to the largest Naval Dental Clinic in the world. My wife applied to the residency closest to Norfolk by way of a non-stop flight, and was accepted. It was a great accomplishment for Sue as the specialty residency was the most sought-after and difficult to get into! We were elated, yet disappointed knowing that we now faced living apart for the next three years.

She and I made the best of it and were able to see each other almost every weekend for the three years. I received cost-ofliving compensation for the Boston area (where Sue was accepted into residency at Tufts University), almost double that of the Norfolk, VA area. This additional money helped cover the monthly flights. Sue also lived with her sister in Boston, which cut down on our living expenses.

I was happy to finally be out of residency and a commissioned Lieutenant dental officer in the US Navy. I practiced a full scope of periodontics, completed an anesthesia rotation at the US Naval hospital in Portsmouth, and became board certified, all on the Navy's dime. In return, they got a board certified specialist.

I won't mislead you; it was not easy at times. I had to spend weeks without my wife, with only my chocolate lab Henry for company, and I didn't make close to the large salaries some of my former classmates were making. What the Navy did give me was tax-free cost-of-living, full medical expenses with no disability, malpractice or life insurance coverage needed, paid boards, and one nice meeting a year (all-expenses paid). I also received some of the best clinical experience in those years. It was similar to a three-year clinical fellowship beyond residency, as I had periodontal mentors at the Naval clinic to discuss cases with, and a full complement of specialists and generalists. Also, my pay grade was actually higher coming into the Navy, as my years of residency counted toward my "time in". It also counted toward promotion, and I was promoted to Lieutenant Commander (O-4) toward the end of my last year. I had multiple opportunities to give lectures at dental meetings and teach Advanced Education in General Dentistry (AEGD) residents where I led the periodontics AEGD program.

I was offered a position to join the Residency Program as an instructor at National Naval Medical Center in Bethesda, Maryland. As I mulled it over, I decided my life with Sue needed to go a different route and settle into a sense of normalcy, like living together. I ultimately turned the instructor position down and moved on to private practice, joining a former co-resident in practice in Hamden, CT.

With all the mockery and head-shaking I got as a dental student upon my decision to join the Navy, I look back on my experience fondly and would do it all over again. I came out of the Navy a better clinician and a better person who developed friendships with those Shipmates I served with. I had no increased debt (in fact I paid much of my residual educational debt off while serving), and ultimately, I came out with the utmost respect for all people who serve in our Armed Forces.

Afterword
Taking the Next Step

So, now what do you do?
I've saved this final chapter for those who have stuck with me to the end of this book. I encourage you to focus on the different aspects of the new marketing chapters I have added to this edition and to begin applying them to your practice.

Upon graduating from dental school, my wife and I had over $200,000 in student loan debt. Sadly, today's average student has much more debt. If you, like most young dentists, are worried about your financial future and want to free yourself of money worries completely and forever, then listen very closely to what I'm about to tell you.

I don't want you to waste the tens of thousands of dollars I've wasted over the years by hiring and then firing consultants with little to nothing to show for it. I've spent the last three years formulating and perfecting a system that has taken my practice from roughly a 47 percent to an 83 percent case acceptance rate. It has also made us the go-to authority practice in our area.

Let me ask you a question.

Do you know your practice numbers by heart? More specifically, do you know what your case acceptance is? Are you constantly tracking it and involving your team to track it as well? The majority of dentists don't.

The bad news is you're not doing it, but the great news is now you know why you should be doing it! Now you can begin to focus on one of the most important aspects of a dental practice ... helping your patients go through with the treatment they need to keep their mouths healthy.

To me, there used to be nothing more frustrating than spending an hour discussing the many problems in Mrs. Jones's mouth, walking her step-by-step through how she acquired gum disease, that it doesn't hurt, how it eats away the bone, and then have her tell me that she'd like to go and "think about it."
Man, did I ever hate hearing "I'll think about it," and early in my dental career, I heard this routinely.

I have always been a slow learner, so it took me a while to figure out that if patients had to think about "it," it was because *I lacked authority to foreclose uncertain pondering*. It was about me, not about "it" — whatever "it" was. It was about me, not them. All MY fault.

I'm now in the process of launching a **New Patient Case Acceptance System** to pre-sell, pre-qualify, and establish expert positioning with patients. And the system can be customized specifically for you and your practice.

Keep in mind ...

This is the exact same system I used to increase my case acceptance rate by 77 percent, from 47 percent to 83 percent ...

And of course, the biggest benefit to you is greater case acceptance with ZERO work on your part. The New Patient Case Acceptance System does all the work for you.

You may be wondering where the idea of offering this system came from. A friend of mine, Craig Garber, who also happens to be one of the top dental copywriters, learned of the system I was using exclusively in my practice to build trust and expert authority status with our patients. He
was the one who told me that I would be doing the dental community a <u>disservice</u> by not sharing my system with other practices.

To be honest with you, I guess dental school teaches us to stay so focused on doing the best we can ourselves that we rarely think about helping others in the process. I'm very thankful that Craig brought this to my attention—because now this system is helping dentists across the country, dentists just like you.

To get more information about this system, simply go to: **www.CaseAcceptanceSystem.com**

If you have any questions about the New Patient Case Acceptance System or anything else in this book, please feel free to call me at my office, **318.998.3027**, or email me directly at **DrJeffreyAnzalone@gmail.com**.